Shaking

Jim Higgins

authorHOUSE®

AuthorHouse™ UK Ltd.
500 Avebury Boulevard
Central Milton Keynes, MK9 2BE
www.authorhouse.co.uk
Phone: 08001974150

First published by AuthorHouse 9/17/2008

ISBN: 978-1-4343-8994-7 (sc)

Printed in the United States of America
Bloomington, Indiana

This book is printed on acid-free paper.

*Dedicated to the memory of
my mother Cathie, brother Thomas,
both died tragically, and Auntie May.*

CONTENTS

Chapter One
BEFORE MY TIME

Annie was born into a large family of fifteen children, whose parents were of Irish descent, and came from County Donegal. They had moved to Glasgow towards the end 1880, and settled in the Anderston district of the city, where Annie was born in 1888.

When she left school, Annie managed to get a job in the local factory, and as jobs were hard get, she thought herself very lucky. She enjoyed her work, and made many friends. Times were hard at the turn of the Century, and her wages helped with the family budget. The Catholic Church and their faith had an important input into the lives of the family. Annie's parents always insisted that the children made their duties. They never missed Mass or Holy Communion, and Confession. Each Lent Annie and her sisters, Mary and Maggie would take all the children to Devotions.

Annie and her older brothers and sisters, along with their friends did enjoy a "Wee night out", and they would go to the dances that were held in the church hall. It was there that met a young seaman, named Johnny, and he came from Port Glasgow, but Glasgow was his home port! After a few dances he asked her out, and it was not long before they fell in love and decided to get married. Being a merchant seaman, it was unfortunately not long before he had to return to sea, his ships would sail the World, and his voyages would take him away for six months or more. When his ship returned to her home port, Johnny would rush to see Annie, and take her for long walks, or they would go to the dancing. They became engaged and began to plan their wedding. Johnny returned to sea, and on his next return home they got married. They had a lovely white wedding in Saint Patrick's Church, all their friends, and members of both families were there, although unlike Annie, the lovely Bride, the Groom came from a very small family only having one sister, Peggy, and both his parents were dead. After spending a few days honeymoon with Annie, Johnny had to return to his ship and sail the seven seas. The year passed by and they had many children and holiday's in Ireland.

After they had rounded up all the children, they had to cross the city to the station to catch the train for Donegal. It was a beautiful journey, but the children were too tired to enjoy it. At the border with the Irish Republic they had to go through the customs. They stayed in Buncrana, where they rented a small cottage. The mothers did all the cooking, washing and cleaning, it was still hard work, even on holiday, but they did not mind as long as the children were enjoying themselves. They enjoyed going on long walks and to the beach, which was nearby. Market day was always a special event, and sometimes the shows came to town. They returned year after year.

After the holiday they went back to work and school and the chores of everyday life. It was "The Depression" and money was in very short supply, however Annie always managed to make ends meet. Social events like a dance or a concert were organized in the church hall. It gave everyone the opportunity to meet old friends and make new one in Anderson "The Talkies" had just started in the picture ball. Everyone was going to see the new "miracle" talking pictures, a film starring Al Jolson, "The Jazz Singer". Everyone went to see it many times. Johnny loved music and was not contented until he had saved up enough money to buy his first wireless. He loved to listen to the music and comedy programmes.

By this time May, the eldest of the family had left school at the age of fourteen. She got a job in the factory of "David Carlaw". It was a printers and printed tickets for the tramcars and buses, and also theatres and dance halls. May always enjoyed her work and made many friends. When she came home from work, after dinner she always had her head in a book. May had to read anything with print on it, much to the annoyance of her mother and father. or Ma and Da as the children would call them.

At the age of fourteen in 1929 Cathie, like May, left school. She, like May, could have stayed on for higher education. The Headmistress would have liked her to go to Our Lady and Saint Francis High School, but again the family needed money, so she also had to get a job in the printers where May worked, and, like May, proved to be a very good worker. May worked in the packing department, and Cathie worked as a cutter in the ticket department, where tramcar, bus and theatre tickets where added luxury of an inside toilet. As soon as Annie heard of this she went straight up to see the factor, to ask him if she could have the house to rent, as her family were growing, and it was becoming very cramped in a single-end (a one apartment house). As Annie always paid her rent on time, the factor decided to let her have the house to rent. The children thought that it was marvellous having their own inside toilet, no more standing out on the landing waiting to spend a penny, or standing behind the outside door waiting for somebody to come out of the toilet on the landing, and rushing out only to find that another neighbour had "beaten you to it"!

The new flat was in a tenement building which had a big backcourt, it was surrounded on all four sides by tenement buildings. It was like a village green, but without grass, or a Maypole. It did have plenty of poles, but they were for the washing lines. In the centre of the backcourt, was a small brick construction. The Middens, where all the rubbish was put to be collected by the council middenmen. The washing lines were used everyday in the summertime by the mothers, who had to stand and do big washings at the kitchen sink, with the sweat running down their faces, as their young children cried at their feet and tugged at their apron. In the winter the washing had to be hung upon the pully to dry. If the pully was in the kitchen the fire in the big black range helped to dry the clothes quickly, but if the pully was in the lobby, the clothes took ages to day.

In the summertime the children enjoyed playing games in the backcourt, and out in the street at the front of the building. They enjoyed playing games like peever (hop-scotch), kick the can, tig, hide and seek. Favourite with the boys was football. The boys put four of their jackets down on the ground for goalposts, and pretended that they were playing for their favourite team, Celtic or Rangers. The girls also liked to play with skipping ropes, and sang wee street-songs, that had been taught to them by their mothers and grannies, sometimes they made up their own songs. In the nice bright summer evenings, the Mammies liked to sit on the back-close steps watching the children play, and do their knitting or darning, or just have a good blether! Some of the mammies liked to join in the games, and would take part in the skipping, kawing the ropes and singing, or sometimes having a skip over the ropes themselves.

Street entertainers came some days when the children were on holiday from school and put on a backcourt concert. Some of the entertainers were extremely talented singers and dancers and there were even magicians and a ventriloquist, who had fearful looking dummies, who sometimes frightened the children. The children and adults liked to make their own entertainment by putting on their own backcourt concerts; dressing up in old clothes and fancy dress, painting their faces, building a stage and singing the popular songs of the day.

The summers seemed long and hot, so hot that the tar melted in the street. A ragman came alone the street with his horse and cart, and there would be some excitement as he would cry out "Any old rags". When he stopped, he exchanged small toys and balloons with the children for old clothes and bedding, and if any woman had rags he gave her cups and plates in exchange. The coalman also came down the street with his horse and cart, and he shouted "coal n' brickets" at the pitch of his voice; Selling it to those who could afford it. Sometimes people bought the coal in the summertime when it was cheap, and stored it in a bunker for the winter, when it would cost a lot more. Their horses always dejaecated in the street leaving a mess for someone to clean-up. Glasgow had three evening newspapers, and the paper-boy came down the street shouting "Times, News, Citizen", the paper cost about a half-penny, so people could buy it and give themselves a good evenings reading. The children also liked to go and play in Kelvingrove Park, which was near-by, because it had a good swing park which the younger children enjoyed. There was also the Kelvingrove Art Gallery, which has some of the World's finest exhibits. The older children liked to go there when the weather was bad.

The highlight of each summer was when Annie and her sisters Mary and Maggie took their families on holiday. They did not have much money, but they managed to save enough to take their families to Ireland, their favourite destination. As their husbands were still at sea the sisters got all the packing done and the children ready. At last the day everyone had been looking forward to had arrived and everyone was so excited and very tired because they they had not slept the previous night. Everyone carried a piece of luggage or a bag of food that they took with them to eat on the ship, which sailed from the Broomilaw in Glasgow down the River Clyde, past Paddy's Milestone, and out into the sea to Northern Ireland. The sail was a strain on Annie and her sisters as the children got very excited, and and they could not sleep because of the noise of the cattle, mooing on the beck below. Daybreak, and it was time to collect all their belongings and disembark, so glad that this part of the journey was over.

After they had rounded up all the children, they had to cross the city to the station to catch the train for Donegal. It was a beautiful journey, but the children were too tired to enjoy it. At the border with the Irish Republic they had to go through the customs. They stayed in Buncrana, where they rented a small cottage. The mothers did all the cooking, washing and cleaning, it was still hard work, even on holiday, but they did not mind as long as the children were enjoying themselves. They enjoyed going on long walks and to the beach, which was nearby. Market days was always a special event, and sometimes the shows came to town, They returned year after year.

After the holiday they went back to work and school and the chores of everyday life. It was "The Depression" and money was in very short supply, however Annie always managed to make ends meet. Social events like a dance or a concert were organized in the church hall. It gave everyone the opportunity to meet old friends and make new once in Anderson "The Talkies" had just started in the picture ball. Everyone was going to see the new "miracle" talking pictures, a film starring Al Jolson, "The Jazz Singer". Everyone went to see it many times. Johnny loved music and was not contented until he had saved up enough money to buy his first wireless. He loved to listen to the music and comedy programmes.

By this time May, the eldest of the family had left school at the age of fourteen. She got a job in the factory of "David Carlaw". It was a printers and printed tickets for the tramcars and buses, and also theatres and dance halls. May always enjoyed her work and made many friends. When she came home from work, after dinner she always had her head in a book.

May had to read anything with print on it, much to the annoyance of her mother and father. or Ma and Da as the children would call them.

At the age of fourteen in 1929 Cathie, like May, left school. She, like May, could have stayed on for higher education. The Headmistress would have liked her to go to Our Lady and Saint Francis High School, but again the family needed money, so she also had to get a job in the printers where May worked, and, like May, proved to be a very good worker. May worked in the packing department, and Cathie worked as a cutter in the ticket department, where tramcar, bus and theatre tickets where printed. Sometimes Cathie would be sent out by Mr. Carlaw to deliver big parcels of tickets. She enjoyed going out in the summertime when it was nice and sunny, but in the winter she got cold and wet in the heavy rain and snow. Once a year they had a works outing. Everyone enjoyed a bus run into the country, or a sail "doon the watter" to Dunoon.

Annie's sisters and brothers lived nearby, always helping each other in the hour of need. If Annie Mary or Maggie were short of money, or ill and they needed money for the doctor, who had to be paid for making a home visit. Sometimes they had to lone each other money to buy a bag of coal, if their husbands wages were late in arriving from the shipping company. Maggie's husband, Charlie was a docker, working in the Glasgow docks nearly always had her money on time. Sometimes the money would be for a bag of coal for the fire in the range in the kitchen. The coal in the fire would cause a lot of soot to go up the lum (chimney), and once or twice a year they would have to get the chimney sweep to clean the lum. Annie and Mary and Maggie hated having this job done as it disrupted their kitchen, everything having to be covered; Annie said to Mary "I wish that we lived in a warn climate, and we would not have to have this job done!" In the winter the smoke from the chimneys caused a lot of fog and smog, which was very bad for peoples health. The fog also made it very difficult to see, and Cathie and May hated coming home from their work in the dark thick fog. "It wont stop you from going out to the dancing" Annie told Cathie, and she continued "It "It wont stop you from smoking, and that cough of your's is also bad for your health, and that goes for you too May". The smog made it very hard to see!

The made many friends at work, the working day was long and the work was hard, but they made the the time pass by talking about their boyfriends and the dancing, also singing the popular songs. Cathie was a very good knitter, and like some of her work-mates, she brought her knitting into work to do at the lunch break and tea breaks. Big Bella told Cathie "You've got gifted hands, I wish that I could knit like that". Cathie's speciality was her shawls, and she always knitted one for her friends if they got married and had a baby. Cathie and Wee Masie also did the girls hair at lunch-time if any of her friends had a date or were going to the dancing. Once or twice a week they would go to the dancing, and dance the waltz, the quick-step and the slow-fox-trot. Sometimes they would get a boy friend, who would walk them home, if they knew them, and if they were late in returning home, Annie was behind the door with the carpet beater (which she normally used to beat a small fireside rug when on the washing line) and hit them with it on the backside as they came in. As Cathie and May arrived home ten minutes late, they received a stroke of the carpet beater across the backside from Annie, who shouted, "Your late", as she administered the stroke of the carpet beater, which was made of cane "ten minutes, your late by ten minutes". "O Ma, you know where we where, and who we were with" said Cathie and May.

Wages were still poor in the printers where May and Cathie worked, however the workers started a holiday club, and put some money from their wages each Friday into the holiday club bank. As it was Glasgow in late 19930's, May and Cathie and their friends knew that they were fortunate to have jobs and be able to save for a holiday with their friends. They managed to save up enough money to go for their weeks' holiday to Ireland. It was May and Cathies' first holiday on their own. They went with s some of their friends from work, who were on their first visit to Ireland, and they made many new. friends with the local Irish community during their stay in Bundoran, and were invited to visit the homes of families, who knew Cathie and May from their previous visits to Dunegal with their mother Annie. During the day they went to the beach when the weather it was dry, and went into the sea to swim, May and Cathie could not swim, and Cathie was really afraid of the water. They took off their shoes and went into paddle their feet in the sea, as the small waves came onto the sandy beach. They got annoyed with Pat and Joe, two boys from the town began to splash them with water, and chase them along the beach just for a laugh; Then Cathie and May, with their friends from work, Bella and Agnes went for long walks in the lovely countryside. It was Bella and Agnes' first visit to Ireland, but as May and Cathie had been many times before, they knew their way around; Once a week, on a Wednesday, the market came to town with the farmers buying and selling their cattle, sheep and pigs, and the farmers wives at the stalls selling their lovely dairy produce, eggs, butter, cheese and their lovely home baking bread, cakes and scones, and jars of jam. There was also a small fair with swings and roundabout's. Cathie and the girls went straight to the fortune teller at the fair. The girls stood in a long queue waiting to have their fortune told, and by the time May and Cathie, Bella and Agnes came out from the fortune tellers tent they were so nervous that they had forgotten half of what the fortune teller had told them. The boys never bothered as they did not believed in it. They had gone for a game of football with local lads, and had got beaten, the score 3-2, and they had to go and buy winners a drink; In the evening of market day they all went to the dance in the village hall, which was a joyous occasion; lovely legs contests, for the girls, dancing contests, and a singing contest. May entered the singing contest, and went up onto the stage with the other contestants, and was seventh to sing into the microphone. May was feeling very nervous as she had never did this before. When it came to May's turn to sing, she stood at the microphone, and after a nervous start, she began to enjoy her favourite little song, and the band joined in as May sang "Kathleen, so fair and bright, star of morning, star of night. At the end of her song, May got a good round of applause, but she did not win the contest, but came third and received a concillation prize of a box of Irish linen hankies. The weeks holiday went in so quickly, Or "Just flew in" as May and Cathie would say. At the end of their holiday they had to get all their packing done for their journey home. They always dreaded going through the customs with their cigarettes and other goods which they had purchased in the Republic of Ireland because they were cheaper to buy there than in the U.K. A long journey home by train and ship was in front of them. Their parents were glad to see them home safe and sound, and to hear their stories, and receive the nice presents which May and Cathie had brought home. Early to bed that evening, for the next day, they had to return to their work. May and Cathie were not looking forward to it. "We wish that the holiday would have gone on for ever" the girls told Annie. "unfortunately, no work, no play" was Annies' reply. The following day, Monday, and it was back to the old routine at work, and a very long hard day at the printers. Cathie and May, Bella and Agnes exchanged stories with their workmates about how they had enjoyed their holiday, and said that they would be returning to Donegal next year. A they talked of their holiday, Cathie cut her finger on the sharp edge of sheets of paper as she was cutting it on a guillotine, and had to go to the ambulance room to have it attended too, May said, "Well, it did make the first day back at work go in quicker. Before they went home, feeling very tired after their first day back at work, Big Bella asked Mick, the packer, when he was restarting the holiday club for next year, as she was anxious to have enough money saved for next years holiday!

The younger of Annie and Johnny's children, Tommy, Frank, Ellen, Margaret and James were growing up fast, and growing out of their clothes and shoes, which Annie had to renew at great expense. Money was in short supply in the household, as it as in every working-class household in the 1 930's. Annie managed to have her family fed and clothed as best she could from Johnny's small earnings! The younger children in the family had their own interests. Tommy was a great football fan. "Celtic Baft", Johnny, coming from Greenock, and a Morton supporter (although he had never been to a match) told him. Tommy liked to play at football down in the backcourt with his pals. Whenever he could get the money. He collected jam jars and beer bottles, and he and his friends took the jam jars to the shops and the empty beer bottles round the pubs, to get money to go to Parkhead to see his beloved team play. The pubs only took their own bottles back, and sometimes the boys had to spend hours going round all the public houses in the area! When ever they could get enough money to go and see a game, they walked to Parkhead to see Celtic. He loved the atmosphere of an "old firm" game when Celtic were playing their arch-rivals Glasgow Rangers. Tickets were like gold dust and very hard to get. May was also a great Celtic supporter and liked to go and see them play accompanied by her cousin Alice, who was also her best pal.

May was also a very good singer, "you've got a rear wee voice hen" her father and friends told her. She could memorize the words of songs in no time. She particularly liked to sing a little Chinese song. After she had sang the song, people would say "God knows how she knows the words". May was also very good at Irish dancing, and danced with her arms straight down by her side, just like an Irish dancing puppet. Father

Lynch, the parish priest at St. Patrick's, organized a lot of dances in the church hall and he loved to attend, he enjoyed chating to the young people and watching them dance. Sometimes he liked to join in and have a dance himself, and tell Cathie and May and their friends some of the many jokes that he knew. Many romances began at the dances in the hall, and would lead to marriage.

Younger brother Frank was also a good singer and pianist, and sang and played in a in a group with four others. They played at dances in the church halls and they played in the church hall for Fr. Lynch. They also played in other dance halls and at concerts. One day Frank came home very excited, as he told Annie and Johnny that the boys had been asked to sing on the radio. Annie was so pleased that she put on her coat and hat and ran round to tell her sisters, Mary and Maggie. Frank was also a good dancer, and liked to go to the dance halls, when he had the money. The local girls loved to be his partner, "he's got a great pair of feet, the best pair on the dance floor" the girls commented. When Tommy heard then say that, he wished that he to had a great pair of feet, not for dancing, but to play for Celtic!

Young Ellen was also a very good singer and dancer, and danced and sang about the house, but in a little one room and kitchen flat, that all she could do as dance up and down the lobby. She longed for the day when she too could go to the dancing! Ellen also loved the movies and she went to the cinema during the school holidays, and spend all day watching the films over and over again. A search party was sent out to look for Ellen. As it got dark, Annie and Johnny, when he was home from the sea, began to worry about Ellen's where-a-bouts, although the knew that she was at the pictures, there were so many cinemas in Glasgow in the 1930's. As it began to get dark the streets were in darkness until the gas-lighter went on his way round the streets lighting up the gas lamps in the streets. Everyone worried until Ellen appeared unconcerned about the worry that she had caused. She told Annie that she had enjoyed the films so much that she stayed in the cinema to watch the films again forgetting bout time, adding that she did not feel hungry. Still unconcerned about the worry that she had caused, Ellen then proceeded to tell Annie all about the films that she had seen, and all about the actors who had stared in the film. She read stories and gossip about the actors in the newspapers.

Margaret was the second youngest of the family. She was a easy going girl with good looks. Johnny's pals in the pub said, "she will grow up to be a model". Then there was James, the baby of the family, and four years younger than Margaret, James was a spoiled child, by the time he was born the older children were working, and there was a lot more money coming into the home. But it was the 1930's, and the recession. People were afraid of losing their jobs. Annie and Johnny's family were lucky to escape the worst of the recession. The great shipyards of the River Clyde and the factories of Glasgow, like the rest of Britain, were cutting their work-forces. Some people were left destitute.

Chapter Two
A Good Move

The City of Glasgow was expanding its boundaries, and the Glasgow Corporation Housing Department was building new houses on the perimeter of the city. Annie and Johnny went up to the offices and put their names on the waiting list for a new house, as did Annie's sisters. The houses were being built in places like Scotstoun, Knightswood and Yoker, where Annie thought that would be desirable for her family to live. Some years had past, it was now 1938, then a letter arrived from the housing department ofering them a house. The following morning Annie and Johnny went up to the office to enquire about the house. Having made their enquiries from the clerk at the counter, they then received the keys of a flat which they were to view. That evening everyone in the family was so excited as the came in from school and work. They all had got washed and changed quickly and had their evening meal, and Annie even left the dirty pots and dishes lying in the kitchen sink, (a thing that she never did). Everyone was so excited as the got on the No.9. tramcar to go and view the house. It seemed a long trip into the countryside. The tramcar ride took them through Partick, Whiteinch and Scotstoun to their destination Blawerthill. As they pass by some lovely green fields and trees, Johnny said to Annie, "this is miles from anywhere". The tramcar soon arrived at their destination, "This is our stop, everybody off" Annie shouted to her family excitedly, as they all got up from their seats and stepped of the tramcar. They walked along the road and around the corner, and pass by little gardens just off the main road, and they saw the beautiful new grey building gleaming in the sun. The whole family fell in love with it. They went into the lovely painted close "It smells so clean and fresh", remarked Annie. Up the first flight of stairs, the came to the main door of the flat that they were to view. Johnny's hands were shaking as he put the key in the lock and turned. As the door opened they could not believe their eyes as they saw the big long lobby in front of them. It led to an enormous livingroom, four bedrooms, a lovely bathroom and a kitchenette which had two sinks, with a place in between for a ringer for ringing out the clothes, and there was also a large steel boiler in the corner for boiling the clothes. "It would also be ideal for boiling water for baths in the summertime, when the fire in the livingroom would not be lit" said Cathie. The kitchenette also had a big black stove set in the wall, "back to back" with the fire in the livingroom. The boiler in between heated the water for washing and baths when the livingroom fire was lit. Ellen went first to see the bathroom at the end of the lobby. "Its lovely, I'll be able to have a bath every day or once a week". The bathroom had a toilet pan, wash-hand basin and the luxury of a big white bath. They all thought of the pleasure of lying in a lovely hot bath every day or once a week, as there were nine of them. The four bedrooms were of ample size, and everyone decided what bedroom they would have. The three boys in one room, two girls in each of the other rooms and Ma and Da in the other, this had been decided there and then. The livingroom was very large with a pantry in one corner for keeping food fresh, and in the other corner there was a nice glass door which opened onto a big veranda. The girls, especialy Ellen and Margaret, thought of sitting on the veranda getting a nice tan in the summertime; The house was just off the main road and from the varanda they could see the tramcar stop, and people coming and going; There was also some small shops across the road, which Annie thought an advantage. Annie and Johnny and their family were overwhelmed, and decided there and then to take the house. May and Cathie then had to think about the time and expense of travelling to their work in Anderston, but thought that it would be worth the time and expense to have more room at home.

The next morning Annie and Johnny returned to the Housing Department to inform them that they would take the house, and Johnny signed the missive and received the keys to their new home. They moved a few weeks later. Annie had been saving some money, not very much, and had managed to buy some extra furniture, linoleum and curtains that they would need. "Rome was'nt built in a day, it will take time to get everything that we need and want", said Annie. After they had moved, they soon got settled in, and got to know their new neighbours. There were another five large families living up the close. The Clydebank Co-operative Society had built a new block of shops down the road at Kingsway. Annie joined, and had a good "dividend book", once a quarter. As Annie spent a lot of money at the Co-op, and she received a good dividend, which she used to buy things that she needed for the home, or school clothes for the children. Monty their cat soon got used to his new surroundings, and would go for a walk along the edge of the veranda He lost his balance twice and fell into the downstairs neighbours garden, and lost at least a couple of his nine lives!

Sunday Mass was held in Spiers Hall in Langholm Street, and a new priest had been apionted to start a new parish. Annie was always on hand to help raise funds to building a new chapel. But it took many, many years of funding, before they could afford to build a church!

The family had settled happily in their new home. Tommy had got a job in the "Albion Motors" works, which was just along the road. He was delighted that he did not have to travel to work like May and Cathie. Frank, his younger brother, and fourth in the family got a job in a warehouse in the city centre, and he, like his two elder sisters would have to travel to work. Ellen, left school one year later and got a job in the giant "Singer Sewing Machine" factory in Clydebank, which employed thousands. It even had its own train station. It was just a tramcar ride from home to Singers for Ellen, who made many friends in her work-place. Some weeks she would have to work shifts. As she loved dancing, she meet her friends and went dancing in the Glasgow city centre ballrooms. When she returned home in the evening, that's all that she would talk about, the dancing. Telling Annie and Johnny, and anyone in the family who would listen to her. Ellen danced round the dining table in the living-room demonstrating the steps to the different dances which she had learned. The two youngest children Margaret and James attended Saint Paul's School in Whiteinch, the nearest.

The newspapers were reporting disturbing news. Hitler had come to power in Germany as leader of the Nazi party, and there was talk on the wireless of war in Europe. Shelters were being built in the backcourts as a precaution! Then the fearful day came. As Annie and Johnny tuned into the old battery wireless, which they had got from a friend, Churchill stated that war had been declared, and that Great Britain was at war with Germany. Everyone was sad and worried when the call-up papers started to arrive through the letter boxes. Young men were being told to join one of the armed forces, either the army, navy or the airforce. "Your country need YOU! they were told, and many young women volunteered. Most stayed at home to keep the families together while the men were away fighting the war. Some women went to work in the factories to keep production going. Factories like "Singer Sewing Machines" factory, where young Ellen worked were turned into an ammunition's factory. Ellen worked long shifts, and the work was very hard, as she worked on a lathe and a drilling machine, but the wages were good, and this helped Annie with the housekeeping! May and Cathie and their pals from work continuied in the printers in Anderston, and in the winter they had to come home in the black-out. As the lights had to be switched off incase of an air-raid! Some evenings the girls got fed-up sitting at home reading and knitting, sitting waiting for the sirens to sound a warning of an air-raid, and rushing down to the bomb shelter that had been built in the backcourt,, with the other residents of their building. So some evenings May and Cathie went out to the pictures or the dancing. They would get a number nine or a number sixteen tramcar, "up the town" and come "hame" in the blackout. They were not frightened as they had a lot of friends who had to make the same journey. On the journey home on the tramcar, Wee Bob, who lived up the next close started a "sing-song". Everyone joined in the sing-song, singing their favourite songs! The girls had just got in from the dancing, and Annie was making them a cup of tea in the kitchenette, they were telling Annie all about their night out and having a laugh. The sirens started to sound a warning, during the Clydebank Blitz, for everyone to leave their homes at once and go to the air raid shelters. Everyone left in a hurry, and took what they could, not forgetting Monty the cat. Annie always remembered her house keys, and May, her beloved books. The shelter seemed like a second home, with make-shift beds and a table and chairs. The adults got the children down to sleep for the night, and then tried to get some sleep themselves until the "all-clear" was sounded, and it was safe to return to their homes, if their homes had not been damaged or destroyed in the bombing. Some people could not sleep, like Annie, who took her rosary beads and preyed that her home would not be damaged or destroyed. People worried about what they might find in the morning after a night of bombing. Would they have a home to go to; would they find dead or injured people in the morning? They read, did knitting and needlework, and said their prayers to God that the War would be over soon.

One night during an air-raid a bomb hit a building nearby, and people had been kild. "The poor people, God help them" prayed Annie. The blast from the building had blown Annie's windows in, and the house was covered in glass, and considerable damage was done to Annie's home and others in the building. Everyone rallied round to clean up the terrible mess and destruction. Annie cried into her hands as she said to Johnny, "where do we go from here?". Then she remembered the other poor people, people who a lot worse off, people who had lost everything, their homes, and even their lives. Some of the older members of the family moved back to Anderston to live with Annie's sisters Mary and Maggie, because they thought that it was safer there, and it was also nearer their work and the dancing. May said to Annie, "It is nearer to our work, and it will give you and Da a chance to get the house back into some kind of order". Mary and Maggie had moved back to Anderston before the War, as they did not like living in Scotstoun or Yoker as they thought that it as too far from the city centre. "It is too out of the road, too far from Anderston" they told Annie, who said that she would never leave her new home, unless she was forced too; Cathie and May stayed in Anderston until the repair work in the house had been completed. As it was nearer to their work, the money that they saved on travelling expences, let them go an extra night to the dancing or pictures. They did not have for to walk home in the blackout from the dancing or pictures to Anderston! Annie and Johnny along with the younger members of the family stayed home to look after their belongings, and see that the repair work had been carried out to their satisfaction, and that the house was safe. They still had to spend nights in the air-raid shelter with their neighbours. "I hope to God this will end soon", Annie prayed every night before trying to get some sleep.

Margaret and James the youngest children got evacuated to a farm in Ayrshire. They stayed there for their own safety. They did not like the farmers wife, who was very strict, but they got on well with the farmer and the other children. They missed their parents and asked to return home. Annie was glad to have them back, as she too had missed them.

"The War seem's to go on forever, there seem's to be no end to it" Annie stated as she sat in her kitchenette, reading the reports in her newspapers. Johnny and his sons Tommy and Frank, went to the pictures and saw the newsreels of the War in Britain and Europe, and saw the death and destruction in the cities. Annie cried as news came of the terrible atrocities in the concentration camps in Germany and Poland. "God help those poor people, we think we are having it bad, we are, but not as bad as those poor souls, those poor people have suffered a terrible injustice, God help them" Annie sighed to Johnny.

Everything was rationed. People were getting used to going without things that a couple of years previously they had taken for granted. Everyone had been issued with ration books for different things, one for food, another for clothes. They even had ration books for household goods, furniture, pots and pans. Some people saved up their ration book coupons and sold them to other people for money, or exchanged them for other goods; The tobacconist across the the road sold a cigarette called "Pasha", and it had a terrible smell; Cathie and May and the rest of them who smoked went and bought them when they could not get the brands that they preferred like "Woodbine" and "Capstan", which were in very short supply; Annie did not like them, "They stink the house out, they stink like a stink bomb!" she told them. She preferred Johnny's pipe, which e smoked, when he could get tobacco.

Cathie and May returned home after the repair work on Annie's house had been completed. At the weekends, after a long hard week of going to and coming from their work, sometimes in the "Blackout", they always took their turn to have a nice hot bath, and get ready to go to the pictures or the dancing. May liked the pictures, and Cathie preferred to go to the Dance Halls. If there was not a good film on at the pictures, May went to the dancing too. After they had enjoyed an evening dancing to the big bands of the forties, or one of the local bands and the very good vocalists, they danced their "Fox-trot, Rumba, Quick-step ect.", they headed home. Cathie and May liked to return with their group of friends, either by tramcar (The Caur) or if they could not get a "caur", they had to walk home in the black-out. All the lights went out, and the windows were blacked out before the sirens sounded to alert the people that a German air-raid was about to begin.

One evening, Cathie was asked to dance several dances by a young sailor, who was home on leave from the War. Cathie said to her pals "He seems like a nice fellow, but he can't dance, he's got two left feet". At the end of the evening he asked her if he could see her again and she agreed to meet him in the dancing the following evening. After several meetings at the dancing, he asked her if he could see her home.

Cathie agreed to let the young sailor escort her home at the end of their evening's dancing, and she enjoyed his company ! He took escorted her home, and waited until she was safely up the close to Annie's door, and then he had to make is his way home by returning into the city, then changing onto another "Caur" tramcar to his home in the north of the city. They went out on several occasions after that. They went to the pictures and sat near the back, later on they moved to the back row, were they could "do a bit of winching". They also went to the dancing, although Jimmy was not much of a dancer. They went on long walks to the park and to the cafe for ice cream and iced drinks when the weather was good. Cathie was fond of the young sailor, in fact she knew that she had fallen in love with him, and he felt the same way about her.

Cathie told her parents all about her young sailor. His leave was over, and he had to return to his ship and go back to the War. Before he left, they kissed, and Cathie shed a tear as they said their "Goodbyes" and they agreed to write to each other. Cathie also said that she would pray for his safety and light a candle for him in the chapel.

As the months passed, Cathie thought that her young sailor had forgot all about her. Then one morning a letter arrived for her. Annie put it behind the clock on the mantle-piece in the living-room. As Cathie returned from her work, her Da shouted down the lobby "there is a letter for you, Cathie". She ran up the lobby and into the living-room, and lifted her letter. She opened the envelope and read it over and over again. "Good news" asked Da. "O' yes Da, it's from that nice sailor, Jimmy who took me out". Three weeks later, Cathie received another letter, and another, and she replied to each one.

In the meantime Tommy was working at the Albion Motor works and Frank as a storeman at a firm in Glasgow city centre. Ellen was working in the munitions for the War in the Singer Sewing Machine factory. She had to work shifts, "doing a man's job" the work was very hard! Margaret left school and got a job working on the "Caurs" as a conductress.

Life was going well, even through the War was still on. All the family were working, with the exception of Annie and young James, who was still at school. There was good money coming into the house, and Annie put it to good use, buying new things for the house when she could get the coupons. She saved up all the coupons that she could, and bought some from people who did not want them, or who were glad to get money for them, widow women who had big families to feed! She liked to save for a "rainy day" or buy nice things for the home. She liked the best of bedclothes, always buying new blankets and sheets and pillow-cases for the beds, cooking utensils and other household effects. Johnny left all the choosing and buying for the home to Annie, telling her "you know best, I will leave it to you, you have good taste". Annie knew what he really meant that he could not be bothered, and was not interested. He was quite happy as long as he had his pipe to smoke, and a good book to read, and some money top ut on a "wee line" with the bookie if the horses were running.

Annie had made their home really nice, and a place to be proud of, and her family knew that they could bring their friends home and not be ashamed.

They still got their holidays in Ireland, but because of the War, Annie and her sisters decided to rent a cottage outside St. Andrews in the Kingdom of Fife with her sisters to share and take their children. Everyone helped with the cooking and the washing. The children went to the beach to swim and paddle in the sea as the weather was good most days during their holiday! In the evenings Annie, Mary and Maggie sat at the coal fireside, which they lit if the night air had turned cold, and they told the children ghost stories. James and Margaret and their cousins, Mary and Maggie's youngest children also told some good ghost stories. The week soon passed and it was time to return home.

Johnny spent most of his time sitting in the living-room, either reading the papers or a book, he liked a good book, (May took after her father in that respect!) or listening to the wireless. Annie had saved up enough money to buy a set before the War had begun, and it took pride of place in the living-room.

With a large family to look after, most of Annie's time was spent in the kitchenette in an unrewarding routine of household chores, washing, ironing, cooking, washing floors, polishing, changing five beds. Yes it was an unending round of household chores, "Aye, it's a mans World right enough!" she shouted into the living-room for Johnny to hear. She made a great big pot of soup from a roll of meat, which the butcher kept for her, and she purchased every Saturday morning to make the soup for the weekend and she would make another big pot of soup mid-week if she could get meat. She sent Ellen down to collect it and pay the money, which she had given her. Annie spent a great deal of her time at the stove boiling meat and preparing the vegetables, putting in the peas and barley. She boiled the peas the night before, and everyone loved a cup of hot peas and vinegar when they arrived home late in the evening from the dancing or the pictures. There was always a pile of washing and ironing to be done, but Annie never complained. Cathie gave her mother a helping hand whenever she could,, either cawing the handle of the ringer between the two sinks in the kitchenette, or doing some ironing to help her mother, and May did some of the cooking at the weekends, when she was off work. Annie was always pleased to see Kate and Cissy her good friends and neighbours when they popped in for a "wee blether"; it helped to relieve the monotony.

Annie's health was not good, she had not been feeling well for sometime. But she kept it to herself. However, her health deteriorated, and she lost a lot of weight. Johnny and the girls persuaded her to go and consult Dr. Gallagher. She agreed. She went down to the surgery to see him. Annie knew the doctor well and they had a wee chat. After Dr. Gallagher had examined Annie, he was concerned and told Annie, "I'm sending you to the hospital for tests". Annie thanked him for seeing her and went home feeling a bit worried, but said to herself as she walked up the road, "I'll put my trust in God". The only time that she went out was to Mass on a Sunday morning, no matter how ill she was feeling. She looked like "a right wee lady" with her long white hair tied in a bum at the back. She had a nice black coat and hat which she kept for special occasions, and a fox fur which she wore around her shoulders. Annie did not tell the younger members of her family of her illness. She only told her older sons and daughters, who tried to do help her;

One day, Cathie received a letter from her sailor, in which he informed her that he had been torpedoed in the Mediterranian Sea. He had been taken to hospital in Italy, and due to his injuries would be there for sometime, and he hoped that she would wait for him; They exchanged letters on a regular basis; Some months later he returned home on leave. After going out together almost every night, their love for each other grew even stronger, and Jimmy proposed to Cathie, to which she said "I will have to think about it". After Cathie had given it some thought, her answer was "Yes, I will marry you". After a short leave Jimmy returned to his ship to fight the War.

While Jimmy was away at sea fighting the War, Cathie was busy as work in the printers. She was working all the overtime that she could get, and saving very hard to buy furniture and things that she would need for married life. She still liked a wee night with her friends, and went with them on an occasional night-out to the dancing. Annie and Johnny told Cathie and Jimmy that they could live in one of their rooms if they could not get a place of their own, as flats were very hard to get to rent; Cathie worked very hard for a couple of years and saved up enough money to buy all the furniture that they wanted to make their room into some kind of home. Furniture was very difficult to get, and Cathie had to obtain enough coupons. Cathie had managed to save very hard, and she had enough money and coupons to buy furniture. All the furniture was made of utility wood, it was all that you could get during the War; "You'll be lucky to get anything the way things are at the moment", Da told her. "I'm going to try and get furniture before I am married" Cathie replied. She managed to get bedroom and dinning room furniture. The bedroom furniture consisted of a double bed, a large two door wardrobe and a dressing table with an oblong mirror and a tallboy, which was a chest of drawers. The livingroom furniture consisted of a table and four chairs, and a sidedoard. Cathie got her furniture and it was delivered to the house. She stored it in the room until nearer the time of wedding. She also save dup enough money to buy her wedding outfit, which was a nice grey costume and hat, and she loved her high-heel shoes, as they made her look taller; May and younger brother Frank agreed to be bridesmaid and bestman at the wedding. It was 1940, and they also had to save up their money and coupons to buy their outfits to wear at the wedding.

Although Annie and Johnny had offered to let Cathie and Jimmy stay with them after they got married, Cathie went around some factors offices to try and get a room and kitchen to rent, or she would even take a single-end (a one room flat). She was unsuccessful, as most of the factors in the city had a long waiting list! In the evenings, after she had come home from her work, and had her dinner, Cathie, who was "Always on the go", as Johnny would say, could not get wallpaper or paint, so she decorated the walls of her room with distemper, and used a stapling brush to make a pattern. She was able to purchase linoleum to cover the floor, which she laid herself. "Your a great wee worker" her Ma and Da always told her as they went into the room to see how she was getting on, and to ask her if she wanted to stop working and have a cup of tea. Tommy and Frank went in to ask her "Do you need a hand" or "Needing any help". Cathie replied "No thanks, I'm fine". She was quite happy working on her own, with her thoughts of Jimmy. After she had completed all her work the room was looking beautiful, fresh and clean. She was feeling very pleased with the results of her hard work. Especially when her Ma and Da said, "You have done a really good job there, Cathie, Jimmy will be very pleased". "I hope so", Cathie replied.

Jimmy had two older sisters and one brother. Amy, a sister had been left two shops, in the will of an old aunt. She had sold them after she had got married and moved to live in England. The other sister and brother lived in the family home of their parents, who were dead; Cathie had met them, and had visited their home in the north of Glasgow, and they enjoyed many a good evening in each others company, playing cards, and having a "wee sing-song". Everyone was invited to the wedding. Jimmy came home on leave, and the day of the wedding had arrived. Jimmy was feeling "a bit under the weather", "Anyone know a cure for a hangover?" he asked. He was really ill as a result of his stag night the previous evening! Cathie had her "Bottling" or "Hen night" with her sisters and her pals from work. Bella and Ina got her dressed up with fancy dress and her face painted. Cathie shouted, "I feel more like a clown than a bride to be" as they took her around all the streets singing and dancing as they went along the road, in and out of the pubs. They put a chanty "chamber pot" and men had to put money in it for luck, as the girls sang and banged their pots and pans, and shouted "Hard-up, your money for a kiss". The men put money in the chanty "chamber pot" for luck and Cathie had to give them a kiss. Some of the old men in the pubs were stinking of drink, and slavering at the mouth, and Cathie had to kiss them. This made Cathie feel sick as she nor May or their friends did not drink.

The next day, was their big day, Cathie and Jimmy's wedding day, the happiest day of their lives! Cathie wakened up early after a restless night, she told Annie and May "I did not sleep much, I tost and turned all night"! "Wedding nerves, dont worry everything will be alright" said Annie in a reasurring voice. They got ready, Cathie had nothing to eat, just a cup of tea. It was a morning service so Cathie had not long to wait until the car arrived to take her and Johnny, her beloved Da to the chapel. The happy couple got married in the sacristy of the chapel in a short service because Jimmy was an non Catholic. After father Kelly had congratulated them and they had signed the register they left Saint Paul's Church to be sprinkled with confetti as they left to taxi with the bridesmaid, May and bestman Frank to accompany the bride and groom to a restaurant in the city centre for their wedding breakfast.

In the evening Annie and Johnny arranged a small family party in the livingroom of their home. Members of both families attended, and everyone had a great time. There was plenty to eat, and just enough drink for the men to have a wee half. Annie did not like drink in her home, however she made an exception on on special occasions, but only for men. Any of the women who wanted a wee sherry or a wee hauf, had to go into one of the other rooms for a "quick swally" (a quick drink) when Annie and her older sister Mary who ruled the family, and was very strict were not looking.

After everyone had had plenty to eat from the lovely buffet, which Annie had preperd with the help of Mary, they got up to "do a wee turn" (do their party piece) either singing their favourite song usualy the only one that they knew, or reciting a poem. Old Johnny loved it, it was the only time that he could get a wee half in the house, he either respected Annie or was frightened of her! He enjoyed the singing and dancing. May was the star turn, she sang her wee Chinese song. "Ying chang, ying chang, ying chang. . ." and she did the Irish dancing, with her arms straight down by her side and kicking her legs. "Gone yursel, Hen, belt it out, gee it laldy" clapped the guests. May certainly was the star turn:

The following morning the happy couple set off on their honeymoon, they travelled by train to spend a week in Killin in Perthshire. Jimmy's sister and her baby daughter were evacuated there, and they lived with her for their weeks honeymoon. They enjoyed going to the pubs and playing darts with the locals, and Cathie, who had never played darts before astonished everyone by winning some games. They went for long walks along the river bank, and stopped to watch the salmon leap over the falls on the River Dochart. As Cathie loved dancing, they went to the weekly dance in the village hall and ceilidh in the bar of the hotel. When the locals heard that Cathie and Jimmy were on their honeymoon,they had a good laugh at their expense saying"What are you doing here ? you should be in your bed at this time of night!".

The week "flew in" and they had to return home. They thanked Jimmy's sister. and kissed her and her daughter Davina, and thanked them for their hospitality before catching their train to return to Glasgow. Cathie had to return to her work, and Jimmy had to return to his ship and set sail for the War.

Cathie carried on working until near the end of 1943, nearly three years after their wedding. During that time two of Cathie's brothers, Tommy and Frank announced their intention to marry. Tommy had met and tallen in love with Molly a girl from Partick at the football match, and like himself was a great Celtic supporter, and they both had a great love for films and going to the cinema. Being a very good dancer. Frank liked to go to the dance halls whenever he could, and he was always pleased when he got a good dance partner, who could dance the right steps. One evening, Frank asked a lovely young girl to dance. He was enchanted by her looks and her movement on the dance steps on the dance floor. They danced many dances that evening, and agreed to meet in the dance hall again, they learned the steps of new dances, and went for a cup of tea in the dance hall cafe. Over the months, they too fell in love, and Frank proposed and they agreed to become partners for life!

Annie's health was still causing concern, and Johnny decided to spend more time with his wife. They were a very happy couple, and always liked to do as much as they could to help their children. Annie always said to Johnny "Our children are our gift from God" to which Johnny replied "are you sure they are no a gift from the devil, Annie", to which Annie replied "May God forgive you, Johnny". "I'm only kidding you on, he would tell her.

Johnny noticed a deterioration in Annies health, she was losing weight! "You had better go down and see Dr. Gallagher again", Johnny told her and he continued, "Annie, I am not going back to sea. I've spent most of my life in the Merchant Navy, sailing around the World for months at a time. East, West, homes best. At my time of life, I want to enjoy my home and family with you. I'm getting too old". Annie replied "If that is how you feel Johnny, we'll manage. I just wish God would answer our prayers and end this awful War !" When the girls and boys returned home from their work and school, Johnny informed them that he was not returning to sea. Johnny stayed at home, but he soon found that getting another job at his age was almost impossible until one day when he got a job as a hall attendant with the City Corporation, and did his bit to help the War effort at home in 1942.

Chapter Three
A DIFFICULT BIRTH

Two years after they got married, Cathie was pregnant. She was ecstatic when she was told that she was to have her first baby. She hurried home to tell Annie and Johnny and the rest of the family that Dr. Gallagher had confirmed that the result was positive; As soon as she got in the door she went straight into the kitchenette, where Annie was preparing the evening meal, and called Johnny in from the livingroom, where he had been reading and smoking his pipe. "I've got great news for you, you are going to become grandparents, and I'm so very excited" Cathie told them. Ma and Da were delighted with the news, and Cathie hurried into the livingroom to tell the others, but they had heard the excitement, and were coming down the lobby to meet her, and they all shared her joy; May, who was very "soft hearted" gave Cathie a big hug, and began to cry when Cathic told her that she could be the Godmother to the child.

Cathie carried on working at the printers until near the end of her pregnancy. Big Bella, Ina and the rest of her friends at work told Cathie to take it easy, and not to lift anything heavy. All of her friends got their knitting needles and wool and brought them to work. At lunchtime and at the tea breaks they got their knitting out and began to knot. May was good at knitting bootees and socks, using three small knitting needles. As the oldest of the family, May had plenty of practice knitting socks for all her younger sisters and brothers, also her young cusins. The girls took it in turn to sit in the toilet, and knit a couple of rows sitting on the toilet pan! The boss would notice that the lassies were away longer than usual. One day he gave Big Bella a "telling off". After Wully the boss had gone, Big Bella told the other girls "I know what I would like to do with this knitting needle, stick it up his bum!".

Cathie wrote and told Jimmy the good news. The letter took a long time in reaching his ship, which was sailing in the Mediterranian Sea. Cathie waited eagerly for a reply, and when she received it, Jimmy said that he was delighted with her news, and was looking forward to getting home to be with her, but he did not know when that would be; They kept on writing to each other, and making their plans for their future.

Cathie was having problems, the baby was getting very big and heavy. As she was a small woman she had to attend the clinic regularly.

The rest of the family were just as excited as Cathie, and talked about becoming aunties and uncles. Cathie was a good knitter herself, and began knitting a lot of baby clothes, cardigans and a lovely big shawl. As May was good at knitting socks and bootees with three needles, she concentrated on knitting them.

It was a very hard pregnancy for Cathie, she had a lot of morning sickness, "but", she said to Annie "I'll keep on working as long as I can, as I want to get as much money as I can, saved", Annie told her "Watch your health, that baby that you are carrying is getting some size". Cathie kept on working to "near her time" to give birth. Annie and Johnny helped to save up money to buy a new pram for the baby. Annie told Cathie, "you are not getting the pram until after the baby is born, because it is bad luck". The room however was prepared for the arrival of the baby, but like the War, Cathie's pregnancy seemed to go on for ever! In the middle of November in 1943, on a cold wet night Cathie felt that she was going to go into labour. Tommy, was about to leave to go to his work on the night-shift in the Albion Motors. ran to find a telephone to telephone an ambulance. He could not find a public tele-phone that was working. He had to wait until he got to his work and telephone from there. After tele-phoning he had to return home to inform them than an ambulance was on its way, and return to his work. The ambulance took a long time to arrive, and Annie was becoming increasingly concerned about Cathie's condition. "Are you alright. Hen?" Annie would keep asking Cathie, adding "I know what it's like. I know what you are going through. I've had twelve myself. Cathie replied, "I know that Ma. I'm one of them". Just then the ambulance arrived and took Cathie to the hospital in Govan.

It was a very difficult labour. Cathis was in great pain. The labour had gone on for nearly twenty four hours, and there were complications. The doctors and nurses had to act quickly to save the lives of the mother and baby. The doctors were concerned and they finally issued a report line stating that the mother and baby would not live to see the next day. The baby was baptised, James, after his father, and a nurse, Sister Kathleen was his Godmother.

Cathie and her new baby did survive the night, and after a few days, Annie decided to bring them home, and look after them herself, although the doctor and the district nurse would visit! On their arrival home as the ambulance drove to a stop at the front of the close, the neighbours looked down from their verandas to see Cathie and her baby in her arms being carried out of the ambulance on a stretcher into the close and up the stair, and into the house. Everyone was pleased to have them home and kept going into the room to see the new baby, especially May. Auntie May now, who was to have been the baby's Godmother. She was a little disappointed that the baby had been baptised, as she said to Cathie, "I was looking forward to being a Godmother".

All Cathie's relations and friends came to visit her, and to see her new baby, who, it has been decided was to be baptised James after his father. They brought the baby nice presents of clothes and money. "O, Cathie, you have got a lovely wain there with his blond hair. He is a "dead ringer" for Jimmy". Cathie thanked everyone for their presents, and told them that she would put the money in a post office bank account for Jim, for when he is older. "It will give him a wee bank book to start off with, and he can add to it later on".

Some weeks later Cathie received a letter from the hospital stating that because of the injuries sustained at birth the baby had infantile paralysis. The baby was a very bad sleeper and he did not sleep at night. This affected Cathie's health, and Annie told her to go and get a couple of hours sleep during the day. Annie and Johnny, in fact the whole of the family were very attentive to Cathie and wee Jim. They saw to their needs, and both Cathie and Wee Jim got stronger and healthier every day.

Jimmy was still away at sea, but he and Cathie had kept writing. Suddenly the letters stopped arriving, and Cathie became worried. She received a letter stating that Jimmy's ship had been torpedoed, and he had been had been taken to hospital in Italy once again, and that he would be returning home when he recovered and was well enough to travel;

It was decided that the baby should have a proper christening, as the first grandchild was cause for celebration! As arranged, May was to be the baby's Godmother. She carried the baby on the Sunday morning of the christening. It was a very cold December morning in 1943. Wrapped in the new Christening shawl and with the "Christening Piece", (which was a paper bag containing a biscuit and a silver coin, which May would give to the first female that she met for luck. It was an old tradition handed down for generations, and knownone why or when it originated) in her hand, down the stairs, out of the close and across the road to the tram stop, where she met the first female, Jessie, the down-stair neighbours young daughter, who had been to the shop to get cigarettes and the Sunday paper for her father, and handed the Christening piece to her. The tramcar came and May got on and took the baby to the chapel in Clydebank where the baby was baptised "James" after the twelve o'clock Mass. The baby, James cried so much as the priest poured the holy water on his head, that May said that he nearly brought the roof down. James, the youngest of Annie and Johnny's family, said "I am glad that at the age of fourteen I am no longer the baby of the family, and that the new baby, also christened James will be called Jim, that will save confusion!" Annie laid on a very nice family Christening party and everyone enjoyed themselves.

Baby James, now called Jim was growing "bigger by the day", Granny Annie said. At the age of eighteen months he was still unable to walk, and was getting very heavy for Cathie to carry. He was still not sleeping at night, and poor Cathie had styes in her eyes with lack of sleep. Cathie was so proud of her son, and sat by the window with Wee Jim on her knee combing his blond hair, and put a big curl and wave on top. Cathie and Ellen decided to take Jim on holiday to Slago in the Irish Republic, to see if the sea air would make him sleep. They took him on the deck of the ship to get the sea breeze hoping that would make him tired. He did not sleep during the voyage, and Cathie and Ellen agreed that they were really "worn out", and they dreaded the journey to Sligo after they had disembarked. Cathie and Ellen had cousins staying at the same guest house, and they were very pleased to see Patsy and Eddie after their long journey. The fresh air did not make Jim sleep, and everyone took it in turn to take Jim out for a walk in a go-chair, to give Cathie the chance to get a few hours sleep during the day. Patsy told Cathie "O, you look awful, you are looking so tired and thin, Cathie, you could be doing with a good rest. You'll need another holiday when you get home". They took Jim, and Patsy's two sons, John and Edward out for long walks along the Atlantic Ocean shore. They were sure that the fresh air, and the wind and rain would tire Jim out and make him sleepy. They kept him awake during the day, every day, to see if it would make him sleep at night. After they had enjoyed their supper in the dining room, and thanked the landlady Mrs. Cassidy for a lovely meal, Cathie put Jim down for the night, and went to her own bed, hoping that Jim would not waken and went to her own bed. Ellen went out to the dancing, she was a good dancer like Cathie, and liked to go to the local dancing with girls that she had met. Patsy and Eddie's two sons slept all night. After a couple of hours, Jim was "wide awake again" and up for the night. After they returned home from holiday, Cathie took Jim back to see the doctor. "I'm very concerned about Jim". She told Dr. Gallagher, "Jim is still not sleeping at night, and he is very shaky when he tries to walk, and" she continued "his hands are very shaky when he tries to lift something up, and he spills liquid when he lifts up a cup or a spoon. I also notice a twitch on Jim's mouth when he speaks". Seeing Cathie's concern, Dr. Gallagher told Cathie "I will refer Jim to a specialist, I will also give you a prescription for yourself, you could be doing with a tonic". A few weeks later Cathie received an appointment to take Jim to see the specialist. Cathie was feeling nervous and told Annie, "I am concerned about what her might tell me", although she knew from the letter that she had received from the hospital after Jim's birth. "Do not worry too much, Jim might be a ballet dancer as he is walking in his toes" he told her. Cathie was not satisfied, and made an appointment with another specialist, who recommended that Jim should receive physiotherapy and sunray treatment. Cathie agreed to take Jim to a clinic three times a week. Cathie said to May "I will go anywhere, and do all that I can to help my son".

The news that everyone had been praying for, and waiting for, was announced on the wireless. The War had ended, and everyone rejoiced. Germany had surrendered, and there was peace at last. "Thank God, that is over, we are lucky we still have our home. God help the poor people who have lost their home and their love ones" said Annie, the tears rolled down her cheeks as family, friends and neighbours all rejoiced as they heard the news.

The Blitz was over. There were parties in the streets, the flags flew. Vera Lynn sang, as did many others. The people sang and danced and were very happy. Many other people were very sad as they had lost love-ones in the War abroad, and in the Blitz at home.

As time passed, the servicemen and women began to return home and get demobbed, getting their demob suits; Some of the men talked of their experiences in the War. They talked of the terrible sights that they had seen, and their personal experiences. Annie's sister and her husband, Auntie Maggie and Uncle Charlie liked to give parties for the servicemen and servicewomen, as they returned home from the War. People had "Welcome Home Parties", and they were very popular. Auntie Maggie and Uncle Charlie had a lovely big front room, in which they had an upright piano on which someone would play the popular songs. With a glass of beer or a wee dram the party goers stood around the piano to sing. Others would take to the floor and have a wee dance. Cathie got on well with her Auntie Maggie, and she and Uncle Charlie were always glad to see Cathie and Wee Jim, Cathie liked to take him everywhere. Jim was always the star attraction with the young ladies, who liked to nurse him on their knee.

Jim was two years old, and he was sitting in his cot playing with his toys the day his father returned home from the War. It was the first time Jimmy had seen his first born child. There was a striking resemblance. Jim took one look at his father and said "Get that man out of here" from that moment they took an instant dislike to each other.

After he was demobbed, Jimmy got a job as a slater and plasterer. Cathie and Jimmy got on very well, and they were the "Happy Family". Cathie was so proud of Wee Jim, and she took him round to visit all her friends and relations. Also up to her old work "Carlaw the Printers" to see her old workmates.

Cathie and Jimmy with Wee Jim settled in their room in Ma and Da's house quite well as a happy family for a time. After some months had passed, Jimmy began to go out drinking, meeting people in the pub and getting drunk. Then either forgetting to come home, and going to a friends home, causing her to worry, or going off to the football without telling her, and coming home drunk. "Did you forget the road home, your dinner is ruined" Cathie told him. She hated making a good meal, and seeing it go to waste. His behaviour caused arguments between them.

The almost constant arguing between Cathie and Jimmy was having an adverse effect on Jim's health. It was making him very nervous. Cathie was very concerned, and she took Jim to attend The Scottish Physiotherpy Hospital three days a week. There Jim received physio and sun-ray treatment. Jim enjoyed going for his treatment, and got on well with the staff, and the football players from teams in and around Glasgow, who also attended for treatment on their legs. They would always ask Jim how he was getting on, "How's it go'n, wee man"? they asked him. Jim liked the exercises, but he did not enjoy being stripped naked and sitting under the sunray lamp. Cathie had great faith in the treatment and faith in God. She took Jim to the clinic for his treatment summer and winter, and in all kinds of weather, hail, rain and snow. Everyone admired her, and her neighbour, Cissy MacPhee, told her "I don't know how you manage to go there three times a week, I would not have the stamina". Cathie's great faith in the treatment, and also faith in God. Like Annie and May and many others they prayed to God that the treatment would help Jim. In the summertime, if the weather was good, Cathie and May took Jim to the Church and grotto at Carfin. Jim enjoyed it as they walked around the grounds and stopped at the different statues to pray. Jim also liked going into the tearoom for a drink and something to eat. Cathie and May were always dying for a cigarette, and could not wait to get a "fag lit for a smoke", then they made their way home and Cathie said to May, "I hope that the fresh air will make Jim sleep tonight".

Margaret, the youngest sister of the family had finished her schooling, and was trying different firms to see if she could get employment. One day she went for an interview, and got a job in the Albion Motors factory. She worked in a department called "Kiddies Corner" where the new starts who were school leavers worked. After a while she left saying that she did not like it; Annie and Johnny "gave her hell", "You just can't walk in and out of jobs just because you don't like them, you are lucky to have a job in the first place" they told her. "You don't need to work in it, and I have handed in my notice, and I am leaving a week on Friday" she told them.

After some weeks of going to the unemployment exchange, Margaret got a job working on the tramcars as a conductress. She liked this job, it was good being out in the open air standing on the open platform of the "caur" (tramcar). She liked the job in the summer when it was hot and sunny. Margarets bestfriend Racheal enjoyed going on Margaret's "caur" and standing with her on the platform as Margaret collected fares and gave out the tickets. Rachael laughed as Margaret shouted to the passengers "Come oon, get aff" (come on, get off) as the caur was loaded with passengers at busy periods, when the works or the pictures or pubs came out. Or if there was a big match on between Celtic and Rangers, it was "bloody murder" with the fans in their team colours. Trying to stop fights between the fans and the drunks coming from the pubs was a difficult part of the job. Margaret told her driver Wee Tam. "I can'y handle these drunkin bums". Wee Tam told her "It's all part of the job, hen" as he got police assistance to "sort oot" the drunks. Wee Tam told the police and the inspector about the drunks and the fans fighting as they were escorted from the caur. As the caur got back to normal to continue its journey Wee Tam said to the inspector "Aye, this jobs alright in the summer, but standing on this platform would freeze the balls off a brass monkey in the winter", and he shouted up the caur to Margaret "Are you alright noo, hen, I'll be glad to finish this shift".

Margaret and her best pal Rachael had a great time going to the pictures, and to Whiteinch Park on their days off from work. It was there that they met some teenagers from Yoker. Margaret became friendly with a big boy called John. After a while John "plucked up currage" and asked Margaret to go out with him to the pictures, and they went out with each other on dates on a regular basis and after a few months they fell in love. Margaret and John wanted to get married before John went off to do his national service the following year 1946. Margaret had not taken John to the house, as Annie and Johnny thought that she was too young to marry. Then after meeting John they agreed that the young couple could get married.

Margaret and John were delighted, as they were so much in love. They decided to get married before John had to go off to the Army to begin his national service. Cathie went with them one evening to see the parish priest and make arrangements for the wedding Annie and Johnny told Margaret that she and John could have a room in their home, like Cathie and Jimmy did, until they found a home of their own:

Their wedding took place, and like Cathies, Margaret's wedding was also a short quiet service. Like at Cathie's, Margaret and John also went for a wedding breakfast, and had a party in Annie and Johnny's livingroom in the evening.

A few days after they got married, John had to leave his young bride and go off to the Army to do his National Service. Cathie and Margaret became very close, and Cathie, being twelve years older gave her young sister Margaret advice on married life. Margaret discovered a few months later that she was pregnant. She went into labour in her seventh month and lay on her bed as the contractions began, with Cathie in attendance. Annie looked after wee Jim in the kitchenette. The other members of the family were either out or in the livingroom reading or listening to the wireless. Johnny ran to find a telephone to ask the doctor to come, and May went downstairs to ask Katie, Annie's good friend and neighbour, if she could come up and help Cathie.

Sometime later a young doctor came. He was handsome, the girls thought. He was dressed in his dinner suit, and had left a function to attend the birth of Margaret's first child. The time passed very slowly. Then Cathie came into the kitchenette looking very shocked. Seeing the look on Cathie's face, Annie knew that something was wrong, and she called out "O my God, what's wrong, Cathie"? Cathie was carrying a two or three month undeveloped foetus on a plate. Cathie told Annie that Margaret had given birth to twins, and that the other child was a very small boy and had survived. The young doctor took the foetus away with him, and told Cathie that it would be taken to a laboratory to be studied.

The surviving twin was called John after his father, but he was called Jackie to avoid confusion, as his Daddy and Granda were also called John. Jackie was so small, Annie washed him in her big baking bow in the kitchenette.

Cathie was his Godmother, and they became very close as Jackie grew older. He accompied his Auntie Cathie as she took Jim to the hospitals and clinics for his treatment.

Margaret liked style, and she had bought a "big high pram", and Jackie was a wee lad. He was soon walking and talking, running around the house and "talking like a book". He caused havoc by going into the kitchenette, and when Granny as the boys called Annie was not looking he took a large pot and carried it into the bedroom were Jim was asleep in bed, Jackie lifted the pot high above his head, and brought it down hard, hitting Jim on the head with it. The whole household heard the thud, and ran into the room to see what had happened. The following morning Jim had a big lump on his head, and Cathie took him to see the doctor, saying "I'm never away from the doctor with this boy". This caused a little friction between Cathie and Margaret. Cathie shouting at Margaret "Why don't you look after your wee boy?" However, they soon made their peace.

There were always differences of opinion between different members of the family, as there is in every family. It was always left to Annie to keep the peace. Johnny did not "bother his hat", he just left it to Annie to settle disputes.

Jim was not "a wee angel", he also got up to mischief. For example, one day when Annie was sewing buttons on a shirt for young James, who liked to wear this particular shirt when he was going out pals to "chat-up the talent", Annie left the scissors on the table, and went into the kitchenette to make herself a cup of tea. While she was out of the room, Jim took the scissors from the table and cut off Monty the cat's whiskers. Annie did not notice what Jim did to the cat. Sometime later Johnny returned home from the pub, where he had been collecting lines for the bookie. Granda Johnny came straight into the livingroom to switch on the wireless. There lying on Granda's favourite chair by the fire was Monty the cat, whiskerless. it was the first thing that Granda noticed, and he shouted "What the hell has happened to Monty, where are his whiskers ?" Granny came running in to see what all the commotion was about; Granda had "blown a fuse", and Jim had to own-up that he was the culprit.

The next morning, Granda was sitting in the livingroom waiting for his breakfast, and reading the morning papers. He was studying the form for the horse racing, and writing out his line, as he liked a wee bet on the "Gee Gees", as he called the horses. "Uch, it gives him a wee interest, but he is never lucky, and if he is, he dosn't say so!" As Granda sat with the newspaper held up between his arms studying form, Jim came charging into the room, as if he was a knight on a horse and charged into the newspaper tearing it down the middle. This nearly gave Granda another heart attack, and he had still not forgiven Jim for what he had done to Monty the cat. "Do you know that the cat could get its head stuck down a hole, without its whiskers" he shouted at Jim, who turned on his heels and made a retreat into the lobby.

Although the War had finished, some things in the shops were still on ration, and the adults saved their sweetie rations for Jim and Jackie. Cathie took the two boys to the cafe across the road to see what sweets they could buy with their rations. As soon as the boys got their bag of sweets and took them home, Margaret and Ellen had their hand in the bag to see if they could get some sweets. The boys started to shout "they are stealing our sweets". On Saturday Auntie May and her cousin, also called May, took Jim to a gala day fete in a convent. As they walked around the grounds they stopped at a tombola stall and the two May's bought some tickets. They were very lucky, "Well , Jim was very lucky" Auntie May said, as they won him a wooden tank, which he pulled with a string, and a lovely rabbit with a red velvet carrot in its paws. Jim loved the rabbit, but after that when he heard people talk about eating rabbet stew it made him feel sick, and he felt sorry for the poor rabbit. Jim spent the remainder of the weekend playing with his rabbit and tank. Jim sat happily on top of the tank as his Uncle James, the youngest of the family pulled him up and down the lobby. Uncle James was enjoying himself as much as wee Jim, it had been a lovely weekend! Then, on Monday morning, young Uncle James received his "call-up papers" to go and do his two years National Service. He had to go to England for training, before being transfered to serve in Germany. Whilst there, James bought two mouth-organs for Jim and Jackie, and brought them home with him on his first leave. Jim and Jackie could not play a tune on them, they just blew and sucked, making a terrible noise, giving everyone a headache. Cathie, however, was good at playing the mouth-organ and she sat for sometime playing a tune, and trying to teach the boys to play.

Margaret and Frank were also quite musical. Frank could play a few instruments, and was very good at playing the piano. Margaret could also play the piano, and like Frank, she never had a musical lesson. Every time she went into a house with a piano she just had to sit down at the paino stool, lift the piano lid and begin to play;

James also brought home a pen, Jim and Jackie were amazed, as was everyone, when he began to write and did not have to fill the pen with ink. He told the boys that it was a magic pen. It was the first time that they had seen a ballpoint pen. "That's a great thing, every time I write with a pen with a nib I get ink all over the place, I wonder if the the "magic Pen" would be lucky if I wrote my line for the horses" said Johnny.

Jim told Jackie, that he was told that cats had nine lives. Granda had told him that Monty had lost one of his lives. "He has got eight left" Jim said to Jackie, "let's see if it's true". Jim decided to test the theory! He goy Monty up on the ledge of the veranda wall, and push, over he went. "It's true, he has got seven lives left!

They stood and watched the passengers getting on and off the caurs (tramcars) and looked to see if they had any visitors coming. In the winter Jim and Jackie got the snow from the ledge of the veranda and made snowballs and threw them to hit the people passing on the street below. In the summer the adults like to sit out on the varanda and sunbathe to try and get a tan. When Jim saw that his auntie had a low-cut dress on, and saw her cleavage, he said "She has a bum at the front as well as the back"! Well, he wasn't a "wee angel" after all!

May, the eldest of the the family, was a "quiet soul" and when she came home from her work, after she had had her evening meal, She would go the livingroom and sit in her favourite armchair, light up a cigarette and relax reading a good book. She would become so engrossed in the story that she was reading that she read well into the night. One night she read a book through the night, and it was dawn by the time she finished reading. Her mother, Annie told her, "You are a bookworm, May, the house could be falling roundabout you and you would not notice". May had read the book until it was time to get up from her chair and get ready and go to work. "Are you not tired?" asked Cathie, May replied that she was relaxed, and ready to begin a new day at the printers. Her only pleasure in life was a cigarette, and a night out at the pictures. May went two or three times a week with her pal, Alice. If there was a good film on at the local Odeon suitable for children, a comedy or a western, May and Alice took the boys, Jim and Jackie, for a treat.

Ellen loved the dancing, and would go every night of the week, if she had the money, except on a Sunday when they were shut. But she too liked to take the boys out "I'm your Auntie Ellen" she told the boys proudly. They went to visit the Carnival and Circus in the Kelvin Hall at Christmas, and if they had the money they went on more than one occasion. Ellen was just like a "big kid" (in her second childhood) in the Carnival. She said to Jim and Jackie "Come on, and we'll go on all the rides went onto "The Whip", "The Waltzer", "The Ghoste Train" and all the other rides, and they tried their luck at the stalls to try and win a good prize. They always collected a lot of concellation prizes.

Ellen had a very bad temper, and Annie said to her sister Mary "You never know the minute with her, alright one minute, all wrong the next". Ellen and her younger sister, Margaret, were always arguing over something, like make-up or clothes that they had borrowed from each other. One day they were fighting and running around the living room table, and throwing things across the room. Johnny came in and said to them "What's going on ? you are behaving like a couple of wanes" (children).

Ellen took things like old clothes down to the ragman when he came along the street with his horse and cart, shouting "Any old rags, any old rags, delft for rags". Big Bella, from up the stairs said "I'd like to take that old swine of a man of mine down to see what I would get for him! but, no-one else will have him, the drunken sod, no even the ragman" Ellen got enough money for the old clothes from the ragman to go to the dancing. "You take ages getting ready, hurry-up and come out of the bathroom" shouted Johnny, adding "I'm busting to use the toilet". Ellen came out of the bathroom "all dalled up" and ready to go to the dancing, then she got her dance shoes and put them in a bag, and with one look in the mirror, and with the dance shoes under her arm she was off to get the caur (tramcar) up to one of the many dance halls in Glasgow City Centre in the late 1940's. As she left the house, young sister Margaret shouted after her " Ah hope you get a lumber tonight" (a date for this evening).

Ellen met her pals, Wee Sadie and Big Senga, outside the dance hall. Big Senga said "Well lassies, whit's the talent like tonight?" Wee Sadie replied, "there are some nice looking sailors just away in", to which Big Senga replied, "Well maybe your ship will come in tonight, Hen, but you better stay off the port". Ellen said "Come on in, I'm just here to dance", they paid their money and went in. They went straight to the ladies to fix their hair, and get their make-up right. Then they went into the Ballroom and stood by the wall waiting to be asked to dance, and waited and waited, as Big Senga said "What the Hell is keeping them tonight, I'm dying for a dance and nae bloke is gawn'y ask me, and I feel like a bloody wall flower. I've been here that bloody long, I think that I'm gawny take root". Ellen was asked to dance for lots of dances, as she was a good dancer, and she knew the steps of all the dances, The Waltz, The Quick-step and other dances. Wee Sadie caught Ellen's eye and shouted "Gone yursel,hen, you are the best set on the floor. I fancy your partner, he's got a nice wee arse on him". Ellen shouted back "Shut-up you're terrible, so you are, shouting a thing like that". Ellen's partner must have got a fright, because he thanked Ellen for the dance and she never saw him again. After a good night out the girls made their own way home.

Margaret's husband, Big John had finished doing his National Service, and had returned home from the Army, where he had learned to drive. It was good training for him and an advantage having a driving licence. He managed to get a job as a coalman. He drove the coal lorry and delivered bags of coal by carrying bags of coal from the back of his lorry, and carrying it up two or three flights of stairs to put it in the coal bunkers of his customers. Sometimes after carrying the bags of coal up the stairs, his customers said "I'm sorry son, this is ma skint week, and I've no got enough money to pay you, and ma mans no well, can you gee me a bag on tick, son?" Big John felt sorry for them, and said Alright Hen, but I will have to get the money next week". The woman replied "A'right son, it's a'right, I'm going down to the Parish (Social) in the morning, and I hope to get some money from them".

With brothers Tommy and Frank both married, and not living at home, there was now plenty of room in Annie and Johnny's house for both Cathie and Margaret's families. However they dreamed of one day having a home of their own to bring up their own families.

Chapter Four
SADNESS AND HAPPINESS

Cathie fell pregnant with her second child. Both she and Jimmy were pleased, although Cathie said that although she was pleased she was worried after the trouble that she had experienced with Jim's birth. She was also worried about having another child to that "bloody drunken"(at times) husband of hers. She confided in her Maw (Annie). To add to her worries, Jimmy was drinking again, and causing problems. "On top of that, I still have to attend clinics twice or three times a week with Jim to have his treatment, I don't know if I am coming or going; she told Anne.

To add to Cathie's worries, Annie had been taken into the hospital for tests. When the results of the tests were known, Cathie was told that Annie had a tumour in her stomach. Cathie and Da and the rest of the family were very worried, as Annie was sent home from the hospital. The doctors said that there was nothing that they could do for her. Cathie and everyone in the family were devastated.

Cathie bought a new maroon coloured pram for the new baby. The birth had been a lot easier than her first baby. It was another wee boy, which they called Ronnie. The baby was not taking his bottle, and losing weight. Jim was very happy when he was told that he had a new wee baby brother. The happiness did not last, and Wee Jim could not understand when his new wee baby brother died suddenly. Everyone was so sad, but there was more sadness to come.

To help them get over their sadness of the death of baby Ronnie, Cathie and Jimmy decided along with Margaret and Big John, that they should all have a holiday together, and take Jim and Jackie. Big John and Jimmy asked their employers if they could have the Glasgow Fair holiday off work. They looked through the holiday adverts in the newspapers. Jimmy and Big John said that they wanted to go to Ireland on holiday, as they had heard so much about the country from other members of the family. They looked through the adverts, and Cathie saw one that she thought would appeal to them. "Read that, it looks good", she said and asked them all to have a read. "It's just what we are looking for", they all agreed. It was for accommodation in a boarding house, with full board in Mount Charles in County Donegal. Cathie wrote a letter and posted it the following morning enclosing a stamped address envelope for a reply. They received confirmation from the landlady saying that she could accommodate them. "This will give us all something to look forward too" said Margaret. "It might keep that man of mine off the booze if he knows that he will have to save up hard for a holiday" replied Cathie. "Aye, we'll all have to "draw our horns in" and save up really hard for the fare and accommodation" Cathie stated. "Not to mention all the new clothes that we will require", repied Margaret. "Trust you to think of that, you always like the best of style" Cathie stated.

It made no difference, Jimmy was still causing trouble with his drinking. One evening he came home from work "the worst for drink", yet again. His dinner was ruined, after having it reheated, the meat was hard and a bit burnt, and this led to another fight; "If you come home on time for your meals they would be fit to eat" Cathie told him, "and look at the state of you, you drunken swing". She continued "What a waste of money". "Away and haud your tongue woman, and give me peace", replied Jimmy, and then one thing led to another. Poor Annie, who was sitting in the kitchenette with Wee Jim got most of the verbal abuse. "That auld yin's knees are skint with praying, and it won't do her any good". He shouted, so that Annie could hear him, as he went out of the room, where Cathie was putting his meal out on the table. "Come in here and eat your dinner, and shut-up" Cathie shouted at him. His temper got worse. Cathie's temper also got worse, and she lifted a good sugar bowl and threw it at him. Unfortunately it missed the target; "Look what you have made me do, you bloody swine" shouted Cathie, who had a quick temper, and that man had her "a bag of nerves". "That was the beautiful china sugar bowl from the china teaset, with that lovely blue and white pattern, which May gave us as a wedding present", screamed Cathie. By this time Jimmy was in a terrible rage;

Wee Jim was very upset about the sugar bowl broken, because he knew that it was part of a wedding gift. He ran into the kitchenette, crying and shouting to his Granny "Oh Granny, Oh Granny, my Mammy's good sugar bowl has been broken". That was all that was worrying about.

Cathie and Jimmy were always arguing and fighting, and then making up, as they both had quick tempers. Sometimes when wee Jim would not eat his food, Cathie would force him to eat it, and push the spoon into his mouth, which he would try to keep shut. He hated home-made soup, and eggs and custard. Jim said to Cathie "I'm not eating anything that I don't like", and Cathie would reply "If you don't eat that you are getting nothing else to eat until you do, and you will go to bed without anything to eat".

Jimmy and wee Jim did not like each other, and they were quite hostile. Jimmy said to Jim as they were out walking one day. "You walk in front of me and keep your shaking hand in by your side, and keep it turned in the right way, and keep your heel down when you walk". Jim found this very difficult, and he got very upset and began to cry. "You are a big baby" shouted his father, and this made him cry more, as he was only four. This led to more fighting between Cathie and Jimmy. Cathie knew that Jim was responding to the treatment which he was receiving from the clinics that he was attending.

Jim also had trouble with his speech. He could not pronounce the letter V and the sound Th. The V sounded like B, and the Th sounded like F. Cathie noticed this and took Jim to speech therapy classes at the child guidance clinic. It did help him, and Cathie was very pleased, as she wanted to do her best for her son. The speech therapists were very kind and understanding. This helped to put Jim at ease, and this made him more confident, even at this early age.

As Jim and Jackie got older they were allowed to go out to play with the other children in the backcourt. They also played out at the front of the close. Someone in the family would always look out of a window or over the veranda to keep a watchful eye on them. Jim, and when he was old enough, Jackie made many friends, and had some "best pals", Jim even got a girlfriend.

Being three years older than Jackie, and being allowed out to play in the backcourt a few years before Jackie, gave him the advantage of making more friends, both girls and boys. They liked to play lots of different games with their friends. Hide and seek, and Kick the can, were among many of the games that they played. Another popular game was "Chap the door, and run away". The idea was to chap peoples doors and run down the stairs before they opened the door, and not getting caught. Sometimes the children tied a piece of rope or string to the door-handles and then chapped both doors on the landing at the same time, and then ran down the stairs. After Jim told his Mammy about the game, she gave him "a right telling off". She said "Jim, what if there had been an emergency like a fire". Jim admitted that it was both wrong and a daft thing to do, and promised not to do it again.

In the winter, when it was snowing the children got sledges, which they made out of old prams and tea-trays. Jim and Jackie, and James, Ann and Wilma tied rope and heavy string onto the sledges and pulled them up the hill to the old farm, and slid down the hill, having snowball fights on the way up and down. It was great fun. Sometimes they could not stop the sledges, and as they gathered speed going down the hill, they slid into the open door of the old air-raid shelter, which was very dark and scary, and someone would jump out from behind a corner and give the children the "fright of their lives".

The old air-raid shelters were very dark and dirty inside, and always had a smell of smoke coming from the door as often old tramps went inside to light fires. Cathie and Margaret always told their sons not to go into the old shelters, as bad men went into the shelters waiting for children to go in, and would do bad things to them, or even murder them.

At Halloween, Jim and Jackie dressed up in old clothes and their older pals took them round the doors. The older children too, were dressed as guizers and sang or perhaps said a poem after they had chapped a door,, and it was opened. In return they received an apple or nuts or some money. At the end of their guizing the children sat down on the step at the front of their close, and counted the money to see who had made the most. The children always preferred money. Jim and Jackie were very tired when they got home, and told the adults how much they had made. "Can we use the money to go go to the Saturday morning club for children at the Odeon ? Big Sadie and her pal said that they would take us if it was O.K. with you, is it O.K. with you ?" asked the boys. "Aright, if you're good", replied Cathie.

Then, came Christmas. Christmas was the great family event of the year. Annie and Johnny always ordered a big Christmas tree from the Co-operative shop. It was placed at the centre of the livingroom window, and decorated with tinsel and baubles. It looked very pretty.

On Christmas Eve, Jim and Jackie were bathed and put to bed very early. They could not sleep, they were so excited thinking about Santa coming, and what he might bring them. "I wish it was tomorrow morning. Christmas Day" Jim thought, as he lay in bed listening. It was always about then that Jim could hear voices coming from the livingroom. "It's Santa, I can hear him, he has come. I wonder what he has brought us". Jim said to himself as he lay in bed with no intention of going to sleep. Tossing and turning he of course did eventually fall asleep.

Jim and Jackie wakened very early on Christmas morning, and ran up the lobby, straight into the livingroom and over to the tree. "Santa has come, and he has drunk the milk and eaten the fruit cake that we have left him. I hope he gave Rudolf the Red Nose Reindeer a piece of cake", Jackie said. "These boys get far too much", said Granda as he looked around and saw all the presents the boys had got. The boys really were spoiled. They got presents from their parents; Garages, cowboy suits, forts; and story books from their aunties and uncles too.

After all the excitement of Christmas morning, everyone went to Christmas Morning Mass. Jim and Jackie liked to go and visit the crib and see the Baby Jesus, and pray for Annie, their Granny, who was ill.

As they returned home from Mass, the boys met their friends, who were playing out in the street with their gifts which Santa had drought them. Cathie and her sisters prepared the Christmas dinner, which was mostly prepared the night before. After everyone had sat around the livingroom table and had eaten their fill, they could hardly move they had eaten so much. It was a toss of a coin to see who would do the washing-up. The boys played with their toys again, and liked to play even more with the packaging. They also took their toys into show their

Grandparents what they had got as Annie was in bed ill, and Jackie stayed in the room to keep her company.

One week later, it was Ne'erday. Annie and Johnny had gone to their beds. Annie never stayed up for the Bells, as she did not like alcoholic drink; however she did not object to the older men in the household having a wee drink to welcome in the New Year. Jim was allowed to stay up, if he had not fallowen asleep, and to go out onto the veranda and hear the Bells and the ships on the River Clyde sound their funnels and horns to welcome in the New Year. Jimmy got quite drunk, and went out "First Footing" with his piece of coal, black bun and his Ne'erday Bottle, (an old Scottish tradition) and forgot the road back!

Not long after the New Year, Annie was readmitted to the local hospital. After a couple of weeks and many tests, the doctors decided to send her home. There was nothing that they could do to prolong her life, the cancer had spread out of control. Annie came home to die. Jim stood out on the veranda as his Granny was carried on a stretcher out of the ambulance into the close, up the stairs and into the house. He ran, as the ambulancemen carried her into her bed room, and laid Annie on her bed. Still running to see her, "Stop running, Jim, your Granny is very ill". Cathie shouted at him. Granda and the rest of the family went into the bedroom to see her.

It was 1949, and young Jim was about to start school, and Annie gave Cathie money to go down to Clydebank Co-operative and buy Jim a school uniform. Cathie informed her that she would have to wait until she knew which school Jim would be able to attend, before she could buy him new clothes.

Annie's condition deteriorated, and the pain got so hard to bear, the doctor and the district nurse visited every day to administer morphine to ease the pain. For weeks Cathie slept at the bottom of her mothers bed to administer the morphine as instructed, and to comfort Annie in her dying days. Her sisters and brothers and their large families came down to visit her and say the rosary as they knelt around her bed. Annie liked that, and found great comfort in her faith. She liked the visits from the priest, who heard her confession and gave her Holy Communion. The day before she died the priest visited her and she received the last rites of the Catholic Church.

May had contacted the Army to enquire if James, the youngest of Annies family who was stationed in Germany could get compassionate leave as his mother was dying. Mrs. Sinclair, Annies good friend and neighbour, who lived below came up to help Cathie to attend to her mother. Cathie had attended Annie for the night and had fallen asleep at the bottom of the bed, as she had done very night since her mother had returned home from the hospital. Cathie was awakened suddenly, "Are you alright Ma ? Can I get you anything ?" Annie let out a sigh, drew her last breath and died. Cathie saw, what looked like a bright light shine on the wardrobe that stood in the corner of the room.

Choking back tears, Cathie went and wakened the other members of the family to tell them that their Ma had died. Everyone was in beep shock and sorrow, eventhough they had known for sometime that Annie's time on this earth was coming to an end.

Ellen composed herself and ran downstairs to tell Mrs. Sinclear, who came up to the house to see what she could do to help, and help get Annie read for the undertakers. The undertaker arrived shortly afterwards, with the doctor. Annie was put in her coffin with a holy candle by the side. Friends and neighbours came with Mass cards to offer their condolences. That morning Jim and Jackie were told that their Granny had died, and her soul had gone to heaven. Jackie was too young to understand. Jim understood and began to cry, as he had an idea of what death meant, and that he would not see his Granny again. He walked down the long lobby and went into the room where his Granny lay in her coffin. He opened the door and went into the room on his own. He went over to the coffin where Annie lay with her rosary beads in her clasped hands. She looked so white, like a ghost, thought Jim. Just then Cathie came into the room and they both knelt down and said a prayer "Eternal Rest" for Annie, and began to cry, as Jim said "Granny looks like a china doll".

Relatives and friends visited the house to offer their condolences. Jim said to them "My Granny is dead, and I am not scared". The next evening Annie's remains were taken to the chapel, and most of her family and friends were crying. Cathie was so mournful that she could hardly walk. The following morning there was a large congregation at the Requiem Mass. After the Mass, Annie's remains were taken to be laid to rest in a grave in St. Kentigern's Cemetery, where the family had bought a plot of land. Most of the mourners returned to the family home, as they often do after a funeral. For some of them, it was the only time that they saw members of their family and old friends. They had something to eat and drink, and talked about their health, their work, and how their families had grown, and their fond memories of Annie. The menfolk, after a while went to the pub, leaving the women with the "greet'en face wans", to have their "women's talk". At the pub the men talked about the football, and the racing, asking each other if they had backed any winners, or if they had any tips for the next days racing.

It took some time for the family to get over the death of Annie. Life had to go on. It was 1949, Cathie took Jim to enrol him in an "ordinary" school. She tried two of the local schools. The headmistresses said they could not accept him, and that he would have to attend a school for the handicapped. Jim did not understand, and Cathie was very disappointed. She made an appointment with her doctor and wrote to the education authority. The reply stated that Jim had to attend a special school for handicapped children. Jimmy was drinking heavily and fighting with Cathie, he had put Jim into a Protestant school. Cathie obtained a sick line from her doctor and after a period of two weeks he was off sick. Jimmy relented, he wrote a letter to the education authority informing them that he warned his son to receive a Chatholic education, so wee Jim was sent to attend a special school for Catholic handicapped children.

Wee Jim did not understand at first what all the fuss was about, but, he was soon to find out. He did not need a uniform for a start, they did not have uniforms in handicapped schools. He liked the school, and soon settled down. He did not like having to wait for the wee grey special school-bus. Other children saw him standing at the corner waiting, and shouted names at him, and sometimes the bus "took ages" to come, and he arrived late for school. It was terrible in the winter, standing on the corner with no shelter in bad weather, with the wind and rain, and a cold frost, or the snow coming "down in buckets". Once the handicapped children were on the bus, able-bodied children would make fun of them, and sing or shout things like, "O, spot the loonies", and made gestures. They did not realize that most of the handicapped children were more intelligent. Some of the other children, like Jim had to attend clinics twice or three times a week. Cathie was very attentive, and without a word of discontent. She would arrive at the school to collect Jim and take him for his treatment, and if it was in the morning, deliver him back to school in the afternoon to continue his education. Sometimes she took wee Jackie along for company, as he liked to go with his Auntie Cathie for company.

Jim liked being in the infant class, and especially enjoyed working with modelling clay and painting. He was quite good at arithmetic. He liked the sums as they were easier to write down. His writing was becoming a problem, and Jim could not understand why he could not draw a straight line. It would go all wiggley; or his numbers and letters were not nice and straight, like the teacher and most of the other children in the class. Jim still could not understand, why.

The school was staffed by all female teachers, but they were not soft and liked to give pupils who missbehiaved the strap (belt). Jim and his fellow classmates enjoyed the films that the teacher put on, on the old school projector. It was always breaking down and the children would race to the light switch to put the lights on. The films were mostly wild-life and in colour, and others were travelogue's. When the projector broke down the children would begin to shout, until the teacher got her strap out and tell them to be quiet "You are not in a picture hall" she would shout at them and there would be silence.

Jim loved the school dinners, especially the school custard and dumpling, and the mince and tatties. He and his pals always asked for second helpings, which they got. It was always good to get second helpings, and Jim could "eat like a horse", as Cathie always said. But, the macaroni cheese was awful, and he could not eat it he told his mother when he arrived home from school !

Jimmy had not been drinking for months, but, he began drinking heavily again. He and his pals liked to drink rounds of "a hauf pint" (a glass of whiskey and a half pint of beer). They drank the whisky, and then the beer, this was more potent, and made them drunk quicker. Usually on a Friday, pay-day, or after they had been to a football match on a Saturday.

This made life hell for Cathie. He did not come home for his meals that Cathie had cooked for him. Sometimes it was nearly midnight before he arrived home, after spending the evening in the pub. He sat down at the table demanding his dinner on the table at once. Of course, by this time his meal was ruined. Cathie was very angry. Jimmy was so drunk that he could hardly stand up on his feet, "he was steaming" as they say;

One night, Cathie put his dinner on the table, and Jimmy knocked if off. As Cathie was clearing up the mess, Jimmy staggered forward and got struck by a fork on the face, just missing his eye. There was blood everywhere. Jimmy was so drunk that he did not realize what had happened to him. There was blood streaming down his face. Cathie had to go and get him quick medical attention. Everyone thought that this incident would have taught him a lesson. But, a few weeks later, he was out drinking again with his fair-weather friends. He was "a bloody pain in the neck, and would cause a fight in an empty house", Cathie always told him. Sometimes he went straight to the pub from his work on a Friday, and his pay, and drink with his "fair-weather friends", buying them rounds of drink. "God knows where he'll end up" thought Cathie. Sometimes after spending a Saturday lunchtime in the pub. Jimmy sometimes went off to watch a football match if Thistle were playing, or go to Ibrox to see "The Gers" playing. He then did not arrive home until Saturday night, and Cathie was still waiting for her housekeeping to get the weekend messages in. There was always a big argument about this, but even then they always made up.

Jimmy's attitude made wee Jim very nervous. Cathie got very angry. He would make Wee Jim walk in front of him, and shout, "walk steady and straight; keep your heel down; turn your shaky hand and arm around the keep it in by your side", he shouted out, just like a sargent magor. Jim resented this, and the two of them did not get on. He looked on Jim as a "Mammie's boy", not realizing that it was as much his fault, as he did not take Jim anywhere. Cathie told him "you can swim, and if you take Jim to the swimming to learn while he is young, it will be great exercise, and do him the "World of good". Jimmy did not take him. However, he did take Jim to a football match once. Partick Thistle were playing, and Jimmy decided to take Jim to see the match. It was an away game, and they had to travel by train. once they arrived at the ground, Jimmy put Jim down at the front, then Jimmy dissapeared with his pals that he had met in the ground. Jim, after some time on his own was terrified that he would be left in the football ground on his own at the end of the game. But, by the end of the match Jimmy had come back for him. They made their way with the crowd to the station to get the train home. At the station, there was a lot of pushing by the crowd on the platform, and Jim got pushed and nearly fell onto the line in front of an on-coming train. Luckily, someone caught hold of him and pulled him back. This frightening experience put Jim off going to another football match, for a long time.

Uncle Tommy and Auntie Mary liked to visit, and bring their son, John, who was a very clever boy and a very good singer. He liked to sing all the "Top Twenty" hits. He lived with his Granny and Uncle who had bought a radiogram, a new innovation, consisting of a radio and a gramophone. The children thought that it was great, playing ten records, dropping down from an arm onto the turntable. Wee Jim liked to visit and hear all the records being played. john and his uncle listened to the "Top Twenty" records being played on Radio Luxemburge every Sunday night. The following week they would buy one or two of the records that they heard. The program was very hard to hear, as there was always a lot of interference, and the sound would always fad away during a good record. Jim liked Radio Luxemburge for the commercials, like the one for soap powder, which was a "catchy jingle", and the man who said that he could tell you now to win the football pools every week. Jim asked his Daddy, "If he can tell other people how to win the football pools, then, why doesn't he win them himself every week ?" Jim then asked "What do you have to do to win ?" "Just get eight draws, and the top prize of £75,000 is yours, and your rich, and would not have to work for the rest of your life" replied his Daddy.

Jim and Jackie liked to go with Margaret to Harry Hood's record shop in Partick to listen to the records on the earphones. If they liked a one they bought it, and took it to cousin John's home and play it over and over until everyone was tired of listening to it. John was a great Celtic supporter, and his daddy or uncle took him to Parkhead to see all the home games. He especially liked the "Old Firm" game between Celtic and Rangers, and sometimes he was taken to Ibrox for an "Old Firm" match. John was good at naming all the players, and he could tell you what positions they played.

Jim and Jackie liked to visit John's house with their parents. John was a good singer, and he knew the words of lots of songs, and he sang when ever he was asked. Jackie had quite a good voice, but he knew the words of only one song, and was quite shy when he was asked to sing; Jim, on the other hand was "rotten" he could not sing for peanuts, because of his spastic voice. He began to sing "Roll a silver dollar", then forgot the words, or got mixed up, or his voice would fade away, or he would just stop singing, which was good, as he could not sing "for love nor money"!

John's old Granny lay on a pull-down bed-setee in the recess in the kitchen, as she was not in good health. She liked a dram or two, and kept a wee quarter or a half bottle of whisky by the side of her bed as she liked a dram "for medicinal purposes", so to speak; Also a packet of "Willy Woodbine" cigarettes, as she also liked a fag to smoke; Her old pals liked to visit every day, and have her write out a line for the Bookie, who stood at the street corner. They put on a double or a treble bet on the horses, and if they had a win, they bought a "carry out" from the pub, and had an impromptu party. If, however, they lost their money they asked if they could get a "wee tap" (a loan of money) until they got their money from the parish (the department of social security).

The Bookie ran away to hide when the "lookout" (the young man who was watching for the police) shouted "the polis", when the police came around the corner and into the street. The Bookie ran with with the money that he had collected up the close, and up the stairs to his "auld wife's", his mother's single-end. After the "coast was clear" and the race was over, the bookie came back down to the street and paid out the winnings. His "auld wife" was quite lucky on the "gee gee's", as she called the horses.

There were many good parties held in the wee kitchen. Many of them were spontaneous; It was an open door, and Mary her daughter always put on "a good spread". Mary spent most of her time standing at the cooker in the corner, cooking meals for all the visitors. The "poor soul" it was like feeding the 5,000. She always had a big pot of home-made soup, and a pot of mince and tatties on the stove. The kitchen got very hot and steamie with thepaople crowding in to visit the old granny. Eyes began to get nippy with the smoke, as all the "auld yins" (adults) smoked. As they sat around the wee kitchen, sometimes two on a chair, the Granny made them all do their party turn, they either had to sing or say a recitation. There were always some good singers in the company. When it came Cathie's turn to sing, she always sang "Away in the Northlands, there stands a wee hoose"…Halfway through the song, Cathie thought of her mother, and would breakdown and begin to cry.

Cathie, Margaret and their brothers and all their husbands and wives all got on well. They liked to go out for a "wee night" now and again, as they enjoyed each others company. The two unmarried sisters were always pleased to babysit, and look after the children. May and Ellen took the Jim and Jackie to the cinema if the film was not on too late. Sometimes the boys just wanted to go out to the backcourt to play with their pals, until it was time for them to get called up for their beds. Jim and Jackie enjoyed playing out so much, that they did not like going up to the house for meals. They shouted up to the house for a "piece n' jam" to be thrown out of the window in a poke (a paper bag). The children did not go up to the house if they needed the toilet, they went behind the air-raid shelters.

Their cousin Ellenor, always enjoyed her visits to her Granda's house. She just loved to dance with Jim. They danced all round the house to the music from the wireless. Up and down the long lobby, around the dining table, in and out of all the rooms until they were "knackered". Ellenor was a good laugh, and the boys enjoyed her company when she stayed overnight. When she first saw the air-raid shelters, she said "you have a big boat in your back-court", and she called the stones on the ground "chucky stains". Ellenor and the boys liked to sit on the wall at the entrance to the close and tell stories and sing Glasgow street songs, and talk about their holidays, that they all loved.

Jimmy by this time had got another job with a firm of building contractors, and was working as a slater and plasterer. He did not have any papers. He did not serve his apprenticeship, but was good at the trade, and was a very good, hard worker, and he did all the overtime that was going. He worked two nights late, and a Sunday for double time, if Mr. Mills, his boss asked him. However, Jimmy was a wee bit too fond of the "bevy", he liked his drink, he was a bit too fond of it for his own good, said Cathie. After work if he had money in his pocket, he still went for a drink with his workmates, and had a pint or two, or drink until his money was done. On a Friday, pay day, the best day of the week for him, he always went off to the pub after work with his three workmates. Big Tam, Wee Hughie, and the canary Jock, who was called "The Canary" because he was always whistling.

Cathie had been to the fishmongers and got four lovely pieces of fish, and she had dressed it, with fish dressing. Peeled and boiled potatoes with boiled green peas. She had the table all set for Jimmy coming in with his wages, although, being Friday, she knew that if he came home, he would be late and have a drink in him. She made the meal, and then had to reheat it in the over as usual, until the fish was beginning to go hard. "He's later than usual, he has forgotten the road home, and his dinner is ruined, but he will just have to eat it", Cathie said to Jim. Who knew that that meant there was going to be another big fight when his Daddy returned home. Jim replied to his Mammy "I knew he is a bad man coming home drunk and causing arguments"

Chapter Five
WELL-EARNED HOLIDAY

After nearly a year of hard saving, and buying a suitcase and new holiday clothes it was Glasgow Fair Friday, and time to go on holiday. It was the first time that Jimmy and Big John would be holidaying in Ireland. They were very excited about the holiday. They stopped work early, and hurried home. Everyone waited their turn to have a bath. As it was summertime, the fire in the livingroom was not lit. They had to heat the water in the boiler in the kitchenette and carry it into the bathroom in a big big soup pot to fill the bath. Everyone took their turn of filling the boiler and having a bath.

After checking that they had everything packed, they went to bed early for a good nights sleep. They did not sleep very well, as they were excited about the thought of going on holiday. The ship was late in sailing and Jim and Jackie thought that they would not be going on holiday, because of the long wait at the docks at the River Clyde. At last they proceeded up the gangway and onto the ship. As they were sailing steerage, they had to find a good place on the deck of the ship, where they were to spend a very long night. Jim and Jackie were very excited as the ships funnel sounded, anchores away, and the ship set sail.

The mothers got things organized, made-up make shift beds for themselves and the boys, got out sandwiches and a flask of tea for themselves and their husbands, and orange juice for the boys, in case they would get dry or hungary. Jim and Jackie were too excited to think of being hungry as they ran up and down the deck, with the thought of being up all night on the ship as it sailed to sea. Their Daddies took them around the ship to show them the lifeboats and the engine room. They looked out over the rails as their Daddies pointed out the big shipyards that built famous ships like the Queen Mary. Yards like Connell's, Fairfields, Barkley Curls, Yarrows and John Brown's.

Between Dumbarton Rock and out into the Firth of Clyde, the boys went back to their Mammies for something to eat and drink. Then the boys went off again, for a wander around the ship, and Jackie got lost. A search party went out to look for him, and everyone was very worried. He was found to the relief of everyone. As darkness was beginning to fall, and as the ship sailed by Paddy's Milestone, they got their heads down to try and get some sleep. It was impossible to sleep through due to the mooing of the cattle on the deck below.

At daybreak, everyone was glad to see dry land, especially Margaret, who was sea-sick. Once off the ship they continued on their journey by taxi to catch the train to Donegal Town, then by railbus onto Mount Charles, lovely little village, with a short walk to the beach. The boys and their Daddies liked to put on their swimming trunks and go into the water. The stayed at a nice farmhouse. The farmer and his wife had ten children. The older girls assisted their mother in running the guest house, and the boys worked for their father on the farm. The younger children were also expected to help with the work, as they were on holiday from school. Jim and Jackie became very friendly with the younger children, who would come out and play with them, when their mother allowed them too.

There was not much to do in the village. But, there was another family from Glasgow staying at the same guest house, and they became friends. During the day they liked to go for long walks, or if it was dry, down to the sea shore and walk along the beach. If it was not too cold they went in for a swim, or just paddled their feet at the waters edge.

One evening of each week, a travelling picture show visited the village and put up a marquee in a field and put on a film, usually a Cowboy and Indian or a Hollywood musical. Most of the locals loved this event and joined in the action. If it was a cowboy the children would point at the screen with their fingers or toy guns. If the film was a musical, they sang the songs with the actors, and clapped their hands. If it as a rotten film the audience threw things at the screen and shouted and whistled. Jim and Jackie liked this, they found it very exciting. They enjoyed that more than the film.

Market day, once a week was good for a bit of excitement too, with all the buying and selling of the livestock, watching the farmers doing their dealing. The fights after the farm-hands came out of the pubs, after a heavy drinking session were exciting too.

The weekly dance in the village hall was another highlight of the week. It was a real family occasion. All generations attended and danced to a good Irish dance band. Young and old got up onto the floor to join in the dancing. There was also a "go-as-you-please" spot, were people got up onto the stage and "did a turn", as they say. Some of the dancers just loved to get up onto the stage and sing at the microphone.

At the interval, to give the band a rest, the M.C. for the evening organized the competitions. Margaret entered the "lovely legs" competition. The hall attendant hung a clothes line across the stage, over which they hung a blanket to hide the girls bodies apart from their legs. The girls walked across the stage showing only their legs, and Margaret won. Her prize was a pair of nylon stockings. After she was congratulated by the judges, Margaret came down from the stage to receive a big kiss from Big John, who said "Well done, hen". He was feeling so proud of her. After their night out they went back to the boarding house, where the landlady was keeping an eye on Jim and Jackie. The house had no electricity. The landlady was in the kitchen, and by the light if a lamp, she gave them a glass of fresh milk, that had just been milked from the cow, and a slice of her delicious home-made bread. It was still hot, spread with home-made butter. It was all so lovely and fresh, it was so welcoming after a night out.

On another days outing, both families went on a bus trip to Bundoran on the coast. During their journey the enjoyed the lovely landscape. When they arrived they went down to the beach, where they sat and enjoyed the sun and the gentle sea breeze, before the sun was clouded out. The boys put on put on their swimming trunks, and went down to the waters edge for a paddle. Cathie and Margaret joined them, "Salt water is good for your feet" Cathie shouted to Margaret. "The water is very cold", they shouted to the boys. They had taken their buckets and spades, and got down to the hard work of making sand castles. "This will heat us up", Margaret said.

After a couple of hours on the beach, they began to feel hungry. They gathered up their belongings, and found one of Jackie's shoes was missing, and they had to search for half an hour before they found it. Once Jackie had his shoe on they mad their way up to the main street to find a cafe to have a meal before they did some shopping. "I just love going around the gift shops, but you could spend a fortune, if you had one", muttered Cathie. "If you women are going shopping, we will leave you in peace and nip down to the pub for a pint" Jimmy told them. "We are left with the wanes as usual" said Cathie and continued, "One pint, no more, not two or three. I know what you like, once you get the taste of it".

Jim and Jackie got "Fed up" after getting trailed around the shops. "Oh, look at the lovely Irish linen and cigarette lighters" the sisters said to each other. "Mammy, 'm fed-up, and I'm hungry, and I need a wee-wee", Jackie began shouting. They had to finish their shopping and go and find a toilet. "These men are still in the bloody pub drinking, but which one? Margaret, We'll have to go and look for them", said Cathie. Just then the two men came staggering down the road. "What the Hell kept you, you're hauf-cut", Cathie shouted at them. "You spent a lot of money there" said Jimmy as he looked at the bads that Cathie and Margaret wee carrying. "Lovely linen table clothes, lighters and tea towels, at least we have something to show for the money we spent" said Cathie. Just then Jimmy and Big John had to rush behind a wall to relieve themselves before they got on the bus for their return journey to Mount Charles. "We can see where your money went", laughed the girls.

Another Scottish family were staying at the same boarding house, and they all became very friendly. The children played together, and liked to go into the field to ride the horse and pony which the farmer kept there. The other children were a little older than Jim and Jackie, and took took them for long walks through the village. Sometimes they got into trouble, e.g. when they went into the village chapel, and began to play tig, and hide and seek and the priest came out and caught them. He gave them a "right telling off".

It was the last day of their holiday and they had to check their cases. Jim and Jackie had to get the table-cloths rapped round them to get them through the customs. The customs officer came onto the coach and took some of the passengers off to search them before allowing them to continue their journey. They were very tired when they boarded the ship for their return voyage to Glasgow.

The return voyage to Glasgow was very rough, the weather was windy, with heavy rain, it was a very rocky sail indeed; it was also very cold, the families tried to keep warm, as fellow passengers around them were being sea-sick. It was a very, very long night, no one could get to sleep. With everyone being so tired they became short tempered. The ship sailed up the River Clyde and they disembarked at Meadowside Quay. They walked down to Dumbarton Road, and got a number 9 tramcar home. Granda and Aunties May and Ellen were very pleased to see them home, especially the boys who they had missed. The house had been so quiet. Jim and Jackie were pleased to tell them all about their holiday. That night they all went to their bed early and had a really good night's sleep.

The next day the boys went out to play. Jim was especially pleased to see his wee girlfriend, Ann. Jim and Ann got on really well and liked to play at doctors and nurses, and liked to have a wee kiss on the landing, and go and play in each others homes. Jim was walking up the stairs in the close, when he tripped, he was always tripping, he banged his face on the step and split his lip and broke his teeth. Two of the bigger girls Wendy and Jane, got him and took him up to the house. Cathie got a shock when she saw him,, and said, "Oh my God what's happened to him now". She asked someone to go and phone a taxi to come and take them up to Yorkhill Sick Children's Hospital, where he got stitches. Jim enjoyed the ride in the taxi, and was promised a goldfish if he was good. The next day he got the goldfish, after a couple of days the goldfish died, and he was left with the empty bowl. He went off fish after that, even with chips!

The summer holidays of 1949 were finally over and it was back to school for the start of a new term. Jim got a new coat along with other new clothes. Cathie liked to turn him out well. Jim hung the coat up in the cloakroom, which was situated outside the classroom as usual, and it was stolen. At the end of the day the children went out to the cloakroom to get ready to go home on the school bus, and Jim discovered that his new coat had gone. He was in a terribly state. He started to cry and the teacher came running out of the classroom. Miss Mc.Nellis informed the headmistress and a search was made of the school. The coat was never found. Cathie had her suspicions as to who stole the coat, but could not prove it. The school had no insurance cover for stolen items of clothing. The morning were getting colder, especially standing waiting for the school bus, so Cathie had to save up again and buy Jim another coat.

Jim liked to play at football with the boys in the playground. Some of the boys who played needed crutches to get about, and they hit the ball and the other boys on the legs with them. The other boys legs would be black and blue. Most of the other children just stood around the playground watching the football and talking. Some of the girls would get chalk and draw beds on the ground to play peever. Skipping ropes were not allowed. The children went under a big shed at one side of the playground if it was raining, and in the winter when it was snowing, it was very cold, but the children were hardy; The outside toilets were really freezing in the winter. Sometimes the children had to be sent home. Jim and his pals loved that.

Because it was a special school all the children went to the dining hall at 12.30. The cost of dinners was 1/10 (one shilling and ten pence) per week, which was very good value. Jim and Micheal and the two Pats, his pals, and Kathrine, who Jim fancied as a wee girlfriend, all sat at the same table. If their father was working the children paid for their weeks dinner ticket in the classroom on a Monday morning. The children whose fathers were unemployed or deceased got the dinners, and if it was a Holiday of Obligation they had to go to a dinner school in their district to get fed, or they received a packed lunch. one day in the dinning hall while they were having one of their favourite meals, mince and tatties, followed by the delicious custard and dumpling, Jim's wee girlfriend, the school one, said to him, "Jim, why are your hands shaking"? At that point Jim did not know what she was talking about, and said to her "Kathrine, what are you talking about"? she replied "every time you eat anything your your hands shake like jelly,, the peas go flying off your fork, and when you eat your soup, half of the soup goes off the spoon and falls back into the plate before it reaches your mouth."It was at that moment that Jim realized that there was something wrong with him. He said to Kathrine, "am I always like that ? Dose that always happen?" The reply from Kathrine was..."Yes". The reply to both questions changed Jim's life. Before that day he did not realize that he was like that, different in some way. From that day he felt self-cincious eating in the dinning room. If he went out for a meal with his parents or other members of the family he would think back to what was said to him in the school dinning hall. He would tighten up his mussels to try and keep himself from shaking, and the pressure and nerves caused him to break out in a nervous sweat, and the more he tried to stop sweating the more he perspired.

Jim's school work was improving in the class. He was good at sums, and his reading had greatly improved. His writing however, to say the least, terrible. This posed a problem for Miss Docherty. She knew that Jim wrote a good composition, but she could read it , only with great difficulty. The teacher would take Jim out to her desk and stand him at the side and ask him to read out what he had written to her. She knew that Jim could understand his own writing. Miss Docherty would think to herself, "this is pencil, God help us when he goes on to using pen and ink from the old ink well on the corner of the childs' desk". One of the children with a steady hand would have the job of going round each day and filling up the ink pots. The day had arrived for Jim to write with a pen and ink. What a mess. The nib of the pen split in the middle and the ink went everywhere, there was ink on Jim and the blotting paper, than where it should have been on the writing paper. "We will just have to persevere, thought Miss Docherty

Chapter Six
A Fresh Start

The night before Jimmy returned to work, Cathie was delighted to make up this piece (packed lunch). "It will be great to get him out of the house, and from under my feet" Cathie told Margaret. Jimmy returned to work fully recovered. Mr. Miller said, "The next time you have an accident you are out of a job, I can't take chances". Mr. Miller put Jimmy on mainly plastering jobs, but, sometimes he had no alternative but to put Jimmy up on a roof if he was short staffed.

To help him get a fresh start, Jimmy's boss gave him the keys of a wee single-end (a one room house) in Anniesland. It was situated in a row of what used to be miners cottages. As there were no longer miners in the area, anyone could get a house in the square of houses. All the houses were built on three sides of the square and all were on ground level. Jimmy was so excited to get the keys from Mr. Miller, he hurried straight home to tell Cathie his good news. The tramcar ride seemed to take ages as it was the rush hour, with people returning home from their work. With the caur (tramcar) stopping at every stop for what seemed ages, with folk pushing and shoving to get on and off. The driver in the cabin at the front of the tramcar waiting for the conductress to press the bell. The big breasted conductress, with her ticket machine resting on her big breasts shouted to the passengers as they got on and off, "Are you coming on, or getting off, shove-up, move along the passage please, have your fares ready, have you got the right money, all ma change has gone", it went on and on, thought Jimmy. At last the caur (tramcar) arrived at his stop. He got off and ran across the road into the close and up the stair. He put his key into the lock and entered the house. "Your early for a change", said Cathie, "Your tea is not ready yet". "Oh, never mind the tea the noo, I've got some great news for you Cathie". With excitement he started to tell her tat Mr. Miller had given him the keys of a wee single-end up in Anniesland. "Oh, that's smashing, hurry up and get washed and cleaned and I'll have your dinner on the table". Jimmy got ready in a flash, and his mince and tatties soon disappeared from his plate. "A nice wee cup of tea and then we'll go". It was a good evening, so Ellen took Jim and Jackie to the swing park. Cathie couldn't wait to see the house. She lifted they keys from the table and were on their way. As they made their way to the tramcar stop, "Oh, quick, hurry up they shouted at each other, "here's a number one tram coming". The tramcar stopped at the stop and there were a lot of people getting on and off; that gave them time to catch the tramcar. "Two thrupenny ones to Anniesland Garage" they asked the conductress. It was a straight journey, and they soon reached their destination. By this time it was beginning to get dark. They walked round the corner and crossed the street to a row of ex-miners cottages that were all built on ground level. By this time daylight was beginning to fade. They had to hurry to view the single-end, as there was no internal or external light. They quickly walked from the street, into the long dark close, in which there was only one door. Jimmy put the key in the lock and opened the door. But, as the door opened the smell hit them, right in the nose; it was the smell of dampness, dry-rot, and God know what else. "Oh my God the smell, what a stink", said Cathie, "it would knock you down". They went through the main door into a very small lobby, facing them was another door which led into a large room, and this was the house. The sink was black and full of rubbish, and the old fireplace and cooker was likewise. The lighting was by gas mantle, but this did not work. The gas must have been cut off and the fitting needed a new mantle. There was also evidence that mice or rats were in residence. "Should we take it? What do you think?" Jimmy asked Cathie, all in one breath. "Yes, O.K." replied Cathie. It might make him change his ways and stay off the drink, she thought to herself. It might give him the incentive to put some more cash into the home. The next morning

Jimmy told Mr. Miller that they had decided to take the house, and paid one months rent in advance.

The hard work had begun. Cathie was up every day, after seeing Jim off to school. With her overall and her hair in a turban, she was up the road on a number one tramcar, with her brush and shovel, and mop and mop-pail, and soap and detergents, she was a great worker, was Cathie. Jimmy was a good worker too, after he came home from his work and had his dinner, he went up to the single-end and he "got stuck into" the papering and painting.

They got a new white wally sink to replace the dirty old black one, and got his brother-in-law, Bill to put it in, plus a new gas mantle, although it was 1949 and they would have preferred electricity. They managed to save up enough to buy a second-hand cooker, and got Bill to put that in. The one room was big enough to allow Cathie to get her utility furniture, the bed-room and dining-room suites in, and they bought a pair of nice fireside chairs and a nice fireside rug to set he place off. On the days that Cathie did not take Jim to the clinics, she would get the big scissors and trim the wallpaper, the wallpaper had to be trimmed down the edge of each side of the roll. She also got material and made all her own curtains; "Aye, she is a smart-wee wuntin" as people would say.

At last the day of the flitting had arrived. What a transformation. The wee house was looking really lovely, and spick and span. Big John brought his coal lorry, and Cathie's brothers helped with the flitting. They all got the furniture onto the back of the coal lorry, and jumped onto the back or into the cab, and Big John drove up to the house. It did not take them long to go up the road and unload the furniture from the lorry. Cathie made them all a meal and a cup of tea, and Jimmy got a carry-out, and gave the men a drink, a bottle of beer and a wee hauf. After the men had gone, it began to get dark and Cathie got up to switch on the light, forgetting that they did not have electricity. They laughed. Jimmy got his matches and lit the gas mantle, it lit up the room.

Cathie and Jimmy spent the first night on their own, they probably did not sleep much in their new surroundings, and had a night of love and romance. The next day Jim was brought up by his Auntie May. But he told his Mammy that he missed his pals down at his Granda's place. Although he liked his new home, it as a low door, and an outside toilet. The idea of going out to do the toilet seamed to appeal to him. Cathie took Jim along to the general store, which was situated on the corner of the building. She bought him lemonade and sweets, which pleased him, and he got to meet the shopkeeper and his assistants. They were all very nice to Jim. He also got to know some of his new neighbours. It was like living in a small village, everyone knew everyone, although some people did keep to themselves, but not to the point of being antisocial.

The houses were built on three sides of a square, and in the centre there was a large wash-house, which had a big brick chimney. The wash-house was always in use, the women had to take their turn each week. All round the wash-house and the washing greens, allotments were situated. Some of the neighbours looked after them really well. They had built greenhouses, and took a real pride in their gardens, growing vegetables and beautiful flowers.

Cathie liked to take her turn of the wash-house. It was really hard work, gut she did not mind as she liked to keep her washing clean and fresh, "its great for the bed clothes", said Cathie. The sheets and pillow-cases got really white, and the rest of the washing got a lovely fresh smell, she liked to get them out and aired on a good drying day, and have a wee blether to some of the old folk who liked to sit out in their greenhouses just having a read or were fast a sleep half the time. Cathie had a talk with the other women and they agreed that she should be allocated a Tuesday for her turn to use the washhouse. On that morning she would be up bright and early to get the sticks, rolled-up newspaper and some coal into the fire at the bottom of the boiler. She set a light to it with a match and the fire was well lit to boil the water that had been run into the boiler through a tap. She got the breakfast ready, and gave Jimmy his piece and saw him off to work, then she had to get Jim ready for school, and after breakfast they went out to wait for the school bus to pick him up. Then Cathie got on with her household chores, it was an n ever ending cycle of work.

Jim liked to go down to his Granda's house to stay some weekends, as he liked to go out to play with Jackie and their pals and get up to mischief. Sometimes their Auntie May or Auntie Ellen would take them to the pictures. The thing that they liked most of all was to go outside to play. They had a great time looking for wood and old tea chests and any old furniture that they could find. If they could find enough they would build a den. It took them some time to gather up the things that they would need, but once the den was built they would spend hours in it singing and telling ghost stories and this would frighten them and they would be frightened to go home. Jim told stories that terrified the life out of Jackie and the other children; tales of headless giants with their guts hanging out. One night the boys were swinging on the trees up on the hill, they had found a big length of rope and swung it it over the branches of a tree. They tied a knot in the rope and began to swing, taking turns each getting twenty shots, too and fro. They were enjoying themselves so much that they did not notice that it was getting dark. The adults at home were getting worried. As the children began to make their way home, they heard a noise coming from behind the trees. The children looked to see what was happening. One of the older boys shouted "they're shagging, he's having a shag!" The children took a closer look, and saw a man bare bottomed bouncing up and down. The children eventually made their way home. Margaret's husband, Big John, the coalman, smoked roll-up cigarettes and kept his tobacco or shag in a tin with his roll-up papers. Jim heard him say that he was going for shag, and Jim said "you'll have to go behind the trees, take your trousers down and bounce your bum up and down".

Jim got used to travelling by tramcar up and down Annisland Road on his own. At first Cathie was worried, but agreed with Jimmy that Jim needed to get some confidence to go out and face the World on his own. Jim enjoyed getting a penny-half and going up and down on the number one tramcar on his own. Old women would talk to him and ask him, "how old are you? what school do you attend? where do you live?" Jim got to know many of them on his regular journeys. On occasions some of the old ladies would pay his fare, and say to him "just you keep the fare, son, and buy yourself some sweeties". Jim got told not to take money from strangers, but the old women didn't seem like strangers to Jim, more like old friends, and some of them had walking sticks, and could hardly walk. When the tramcar arrived at Jim's stop, he got up to leave the tramcar, and turned around to thank the old ladies. After he had stepped from the tramcar Jim walked down the road and gave the old ladies another wave. As the old ladies were out of sight, Jim went into the corner shop and bought sweets with the penny. The staff and customers in the corner shop would crack jokes with Jim and make him laugh. Then he would go down the street and in the close, knock on the door, and go into the house. Cathie would scold him, saying, "Jim, I told you that sweeties are bad for your teeth, and they will put you off your tea".

Cathie and Jimmy discussed the idea of buying Jim a tricycle, as it would be good exercise for him and strengthen his legs. Jim loved the idea, but Cathie was worried about all the buses that went round the street on their way to Knightswood Garage. But Jimmy talked her round, and she agreed. They saved up enough money to put down a deposit on a Greshin Flyer, which was a lovely tricycle, in Birse the toy shop. They took Jim to try it out, and it was love at first sight; "Oh, yes, please, please can I have it?" pleaded Jim. The deposit was paid, the remainder would be paid by weekly instalments. The tricycle was bought and as soon as it was brought out of the shop Jim jumped on to the saddle and began to pedal as fast as he could. "Slow down !" cried his parents, "Slow down!" It was a long walk home for Cathie and Jimmy. Jim loved every minute of it; along Dumbarton Road, over the hill up Crow Road.

The tricycle had a boot, similar to a car boot on the back between the wheels. It was handy for carrying toys thought Jim. It was also handy for Cathie. "Come to the shops with Mammy to get the messages Jim", and they would go to the Co-operative at Anniesland Cross. Cathie would get some of her groceries in the boot and it saved her from having so much to carry. Jim loved to ride his tricycle around the square of houses, and the gardens and allotments and made many new friends among the old people and children. Jim's favourite friend was old Mr. Hay, who spent most of his time in his garden attending his vegetables, or sitting in his greenhouse. Jim liked old Mr. Hay, who would teach him the names of all the different flowers and plant life. If the weather was bad they would sit in the greenhouse where old Mr. Hay would tell him stories. One day while in the greenhouse Jim asked old Mr. Hay, "Why are your tomatoes green and not red ?" Mr. Hay replied, "I have no red paint". Jim ran home to his mammy and asked her if she had any red paint in the house for old Mr. Hay, as he had as he had ran out of red paint to paint his tomatoes. Everyone laughed, Jim felt very silly.

Old Mr. Hay had a grand-daughter called Pauline, who was a good few years older than Jim, and she decided to take Jim under her wing. Her best friend Emily and she would take Jim on outings to the park on his tricycle, on the good summer evenings, and sometimes they would go for long walks along the canal bank to Maryhill. They looked out for urban wildlife, foxes and badgers and wild cats. They would also pick wild flowers and leaves to take home to press into a book.

The picture hall that they went to was The Vogue in Great Western Road. It was very handy for them, just five minutes walk from their homes. It was a very popular place for entertainment, and sometimes they had to queue to get in, and every now and then you could get disappointed after waiting one hour when the doorman would say just as you were about to go in, "Sorry, house full", and everyone who had been waiting a long time would have to go home disappointed. The girls were wise to this and made a point of getting there early. Pauline would say to Emily, who was always a bit of a slow-coach; "Oh, Hurry, Hurry, Hurry, we don't want to be late". They all loved the Hollywood Musicals, like "Singing in the Rain" starring Gene Kelly; and Judy Garland films, and the comedies with stars like Abbot and Costello, Laural and Hardy, not forgetting Ma and Pa Kettle films, with their daft family. The pictures would give them a good laugh, and they would talk about them for days on end, and sing the songs. When Jim turned on the radio and heard the songs from the Hollywood Musicals it gave him great pleasure. The picture hall had a Saturday mornings children's club. It was always a full house, with very noisy school children, and Jim liked to go. He got used to going on his own as he got a bit older. Cathie would remind him to be careful crossing the busy road, especially looking out for the tramcars on the tramlines that ran along the centre of Great Western Road. The tramcars were powered by electricity from overhead cables. The children liked the cartoons, and the Cowboys and Indian films. The serials were also very popular, the children liked to hear the voice say at the end "to be continued next week" and they could hardly wait to see what was going to happen to the likes of "The Lone Ranger and Tonto"...who would say "Oh Kimosavey", or something like that ! The manager of the cinema ran a lot of good contests for the children to participate in. There was one to see who could keep their yo-yo going up and down on a string the longest; and then there was the Hoola-hoop craze. The contest for the Hoola-hoop was to see which child could keep this circle plastic spinning around their waist for the longest period of time; It was good fun and the winner always got a prize; a book token or a free pass to the picture hall. Some of the contestants were really hopeless, and made fools of themselves. The children in the auditorium would laugh and cheer at their pals if they were good. If, on the other hand, the entrant to the contest was terrible the children would boo and whistle. The manager and his staff also organized talent contests. The children who entered would get up on the stage and sing, or dance or say a wee poem that the teacher had taught them at school. If the contestants, to put it mildly, did not perform very well, Jim and his school pals that he had met would shout "boo, boo, get aff, you're rotten,, you can'ny sing for peanuts, boo" and so it went on. Some wee souls could not take it, and ran off the stage and began to cry. If it was a boy, he got even more abuse. The boys would shout at him "Big baby, big baby, your a big wain, cry baby, cry baby", and so it went on.

It was at the Saturday morning picture club that Jim got his first sight and taste of an ice-lolly. It was a new thing just out, to Jim anyway. He went out to the usherette at the interval and along with his pals, bought this ice-lolly, after waiting in the big queue and returned to his seat. As the lights dimmed, he peeled off the wrapping paper to reveal this red raspberry flavoured piece of ice on a stick. He took one look at it and said to himself "do I like it, do I suck it, or do I bite it"? By this time it was beginning to melt and red coloured ice began to run down his arm, so he was in a terrible state, not to mention a mess when suddenly the bottom half of the lolly fell from the stick and landed on the floor between the seats. Jim felt as if he had been robbed, not to mention his embarrassment, as his wee girlfriend from school was sitting behind him.

Some of the neighbours who lived in the rows of houses beside them were old nags. They did not like children very much and were always complaining about Jim and his pals, who were mostly girls, being on the grass, or standing against their garden gates or fences. If it was not that, the complaining would be about the children playing and making too much noise. Some of the old nags would not let the children live, and Cathie would have to go out and have words with them. Cathie would say to them, "Do you forget that you used to be children yourselves?" Jim had a lot of girls in Anniesland, mostly pals; Christine, Sheila and Betsy and a few boy pals. Although they were always fighting over something, they soon made up, and would go and play in each others homes when the weather was bad. One morning Jim went round to Christine's house to see if she was coming out to play, and her mother asked him to come in. Christine was getting bath in the sink. As she she stood up Jim noticed something was amiss, and called out, "Ah, Christine has lost her willy. It must have dropped off in the sink". Christine's mammy, Edna, could not stop laughing as she dried and got her dressed, and Jim went over to the sink to look down the plug-hole. The two children had something to eat and drink and went out to play on their tricycles with the other children. They would get a telling off from Cathie and Christine's mammy Edna for going out onto the road as there was always the possibility of them getting knocked down by a bus going round to Knightswood Garage. The drivers drove quite fast, and the children would not stand a chance of getting out of the road in time.

The Birrell's sweet and chocolate factory was situated in the next street, which was Munro Place, and as soon as the people who lived in the area opened their front doors they could whiff the smell of chocolate and toffee. It was a lovely smell thought the children, and always made them feel hungry, not for their food, but for sweets. Cathie would tell Jim, who was now six years old, that sweets were bad for his teeth, to which he replied, "I haven't got many to worry about, anyway". But Cathie would explain to him that his first set of teeth would fall out, and that a second set would grow in to replace them in time. She also told him that he could get toothache and would have to go to the dentist and have them pulled out. This eventually happened. One night Jim was up all night in terrible pain. Cathie tied a scarf around his face and gave him a crushed aspirin and hot milk to help him to get to He did not sleep and kept them up all night. The next morning Cathie took Jim to the dentist in Partick. In the waiting room, they had to wait for what seemed ages. It eventually came to Jim's turn to go into the surgery and onto the chair. Jim was shaking like a leaf, more than usual. After the tooth had been extracted, Jim was in a terrible state. The dentist was concerned for Jim, who was still shaking more than usual. Cathie explained that this was normal when Jim was excited. The dentist feeling so sorry for Jim, he gave him a sixpenny piece, to try to calm Jim down. The dentist handed the money to Jim, and Jim threw it back at him, saying, "keep your money, I don't want it, you might need it yourself". Cathie had to take him round the shops to get her shopping done, and Jim had a big scarf wrapped around his face. They eventually got home and Jim had a very light meal, and an early night, although he did not sleep very much.

They had lots of visitors, from old friends, and both sets of in-laws. They hated going to the outside toilet, especially late at night when it was dark. The women and sometimes the men would go in pairs. If it was dark they had to take a torch, and if the torch batteries were done, they had to take a candle and a box of matches. There was no light in either the toilet or the backgreen. Cathie kept the outside toilet spotlessly clean, washing the floor and bowl every day. The door was painted a nice shade of green both inside and out. The walls were white-washed, looking really bright and clean. However it was very cold in the winter and the wind and rain woudl blow under the door making it very, very cold sitting on the pan. The darkness was frightening especially for Cathie when she was on her own. It caused great problems in times of illness. Jim had taken ill with gastro-enteritis, and this caused great problems for Cathie as she had to use sanitary products for Jim. As he got better he was taken down to his Granda's home, which had a bathroom.

Cathie and Jimmy organised a petition to the factors and got most of the occupants of the row of houses to sign it. The petition asked the lighting department it a lamp-post and light could be erected in the back in such a way that the light shone down the close and into the toilet. This was done in due course. They also asked the factor if they could have electricity installed in the single-end. This was also done in due course! Wee Jim was so frightened to go to the toilet in the dark, or during the night that he did a pee in the sink, or in a pail. The coal from the fire had to be brought from the bunker, which was also situated outside in the back, just under the window. A coal-scuttle, which was made of tin or brass, was used to bring the coal in from the bunker. Sometimes they forgot to fill the scuttle for the night and they had to go out in the dark, if the fire was about to go out, and it was very frightening. Sometimes they would look round and think that they could see shadows or figures in the dark. In the winter when it was snowing they had to clear the snow from the top of the bunker. One night Cathie said to Jimmy "I forgot to get the coal in", to which Jimmy replied, "go and get it in yourself", now this she did. She cleared the snow from the top of the bunker and opened the top. She put her hand in to bring out lumps of coal, and out jumped a big rat. Cathie got the fright of her life and gave out a big yell. Jimmy thought that she was being attacked. He ran out to see what had happened. "What the bloody hell are you screaming at, I thought you were being murdered," he shouted at her when he saw that she was alright. She told him what had happened, and they went in with the coal in the scuttle for the fire and Cathie was still shaking like a leaf. By the time they got in the fire was nearly out, and they had to go through the ritual of trying to relight the fire again, by rolling up some old newspapers and putting some sticks on top of the ashes that still had some fire in them in the grate. By this time the house was so cold that it put any idea of sex out of their minds, then again "it might heat us up", said Jimmy...

The single-end was over-run by mice, or maybe baby rats. Cathie got the "environmental health" in, Jimmy plastered up any holes and cracks in the walls that he could fined. But still the rodents kept coming. As Cathie lay awake in the dark listening to the noise of the patter of tiny little feet, as the mice played about, she thought of them swinging on the corner of her long table cloth that she had brought from Ireland. She lay in her bed with an old walking stick of Jimmy's by her side. Tap, tap, tap, she would tap on the side of the bed to frighten them away, but of course this only worked for a short time, and then the mice would return. "There is only one other option for us to try", said Jimmy, "we will have to go to the dog and cat home in Cardonald to see if we can buy a cat, to rid the house of mice". The following Saturday, it was a day that the football was not on, and that's why Jimmy agreed to go. They got a lovely little kitten, and decided to call him "Tibby". Tibby soon got used to his new surroundings, and soon earned his keep by doing the job that he was there for, catching mice. Jim liked to rollup balls of silver paper and wool, and roll them for Tibby to get. The cat also enjoyed this. He caught many mice, and took great pride in running about with them in his mouth.

Although Jimmy worked in the building trade, he had quite a lot of friends who had different trades, plumbers, joiners, and electricians. He asked Peter the electrician, if he would wire up the house, and he would give him a wee back-hander (some money) for doing the job. Peter agreed, and he and a mate came up one weekend and wired up the house. The electric light really brightened the place up. No more smell from the gas mantle. "It fairly shows up the dirt", said Cathie, "we will soon have to get wallpaper and paint and start decorating again. A few weeks later they went to the Electrical Shop, and put the deposit down on a wireless set. It was great to have music in the house, thought Jim, and the comedies made him laugh;

Saturday night at tea tim was always a good exciting time, when almost everyone would tune into their wireless to hear the football results, and check their football pools, and see if they had eight draws to win the jackpot of £75,000 on the pools. They would always dram of what they would do with the money if they won; Granda always said that he would win the pools before he died. Cathie liked to hear the football scores, and would be pleased if Celtic won. Jimmy would be pleased if either Partick Thistle or Rangers won. Cathie would make a lovely dinner for the three of them after Jimmy returned home from the football match. He would usually go to the pub with some people he met, and forget the way home. Cathie and Jim would have their dinner then sit and listen to the wireless, and look at the clock, and, as usual, begin to worry about what state Jimmy would be in when he arrived home. Sometimes, Cathie would say to herself, "Oh, to hell with this, sitting her waiting for him". She would tell Jim to get ready and they would go out to the pictures, or down to spend the night in Granda's.

Sometimes Jimmy would be in so bad a temper when he came home that Cathie and wee Jim would have to run for their lives. The tramcars were off at that time of night, and they would have to walk all the way down Anniesland Road. One night, it was dark and cold and raining very heavily. They were also very frightened as there was no-one to be seen, except the odd strange looking person walking up and down the road. As they walked faster, the stranger would walk faster, as they slowed down, he would slow down. It was a relief when they reached Dumbarton Road with the bright lights from traffic and the occasional shop. They hurried along the road to Granda's house. In the close and up the stairs to the first landing. Cathie knocked on Granda's door, she knocked again, still no answer. Jim battered on the door. This time May came and opened the door and let them in. May knew right away what had happened. She knew Jimmy, and saw that wee Jim was in a terrible state. "I'll make you a cup of tea" she said to Cathie, "get the wain (child) ready and into bed". Jim felt more contented and was soon fast asleep. "I'll have to go back up to the house and get some clothes when Jimmys' at his work" Cathie told May. The next morning being Sunday they got up and had breakfast and then went to Mass.

After he got up, Jimmy got rid of his handover. Jimmy went down to see Cathie, he knew where she was, there was nowhere else, where she could go. "I'm very sorry" he would say, "very, very sorry, it won't happen again". Like lots of other wives Cathie had heard it all before. As usual, Cathie went back to give him another chance. Jim was not taken in, he knew that it would occur again.

Cathie was back with Jimmy to give him another, just one other last chance, after staying away for a couple of weeks. They were very happy for a time. Cathie was a good house keeper and manager, and bedmate. Jim often wondered what that meant. She was really good at making money go round, as she didn't get much from Jimmy's wages. She kept the house nice and clean, and made good meals, and Jimmy liked his grub, and he liked it on the table. Cathie got a piece of meat from the Co-op butcher, and would make a big pot of soup on a Saturday night for the Sunday dinner. When Jimmy came in from the football match, he was always cold, and would say "Ah'm starving" and a big plate or two of Cathie's home made soup would heat him up, and go down a treat, "Oh' leave some for Sunday said Cathie. Wee Jim loved a cup of hot boiled peas in vinegar that Cathie also made with the soup. He would eat them out of the cup with the big spoon, "Oh' that was good, can I please have some more?" he asked his Mammy, he was a well mannered boy.

During the summer, the football closed season, Jimmy could and would stay off the drink for months, and spend time and money with and on his family, and act like a real family man. Cathie and Jimmy would take wee Jim to the two local picture halls, The Vogue and The Gaumont. They could go four times a week if they wished, as each cinema changed its program twice a week. If the weather was good during the Glasgow Fair holiday, and they were not away in Ireland, they would take wee Jim on a sails "Doon the Watter", which was a sail down the River Clyde, to one of the many resorts down the river, places like Dunoon, Rothsey and Millport. Or they would go on a bus run down to Ayr or Saltcoats. Jim's favourite place of entertainment was the zoo. Two of which were in the area, Caulderpark in Glasgow, and Craigend. Jim loved to see all the animals, and go for a ride on the miniature train.

The happiness did not last though, and each time the football season started, so would Jimmy's drinking. It was back to the old trouble of Jimmy not coming home from work with wages on a Friday night until the pubs had closed, with some of Cathie's housekeeping money short, and spent on drink, or coming home from the match on a Saturday night and throwing a "brainstorm".

Cathie and wee Jim never missed Mass. They always went on a Sunday morning and on a holiday of obligation. One day Jimmy, who was a good worker, worked hard, and worked a lot of overtime whenever he was asked, was off work for some reason. Jim was at school, and Jimmy and Cathie had been arguing. Cathie had gone to get some messages at the Co-op and when she returned she found that Jimmy and her holy pictures had gone. This is very strange though Cathie, although she had a good idea what had happened, and she was right. Jimmy had taken them up to the chapel house, chapped the door, and when the housekeeper opened the door, Jimmy threw the pictures in the door saying, "these belong here, and not in my house". The priest came to the door and they exchanged words, then Jimmy went for a drink.

Cathie had a good look around the house, just to make sure, and she found that her picture of Our Lady, and one of the Sacred Heart had gone. She looked in a drawer to find that her rosary beads had also disappeared. Soon Jimmy returned, with a drink in him. "Where are my pictures and my rosary beads ?" asked Cathie. "Where they belong" replied Jimmy, and one thing led to another, and there was a fight between them. Punches were made at both and Jimmy got a hold of Cathie by the hair and pulled her out of the door and all along the stone floor of the close. Cathie was squealing, her stockings were torn, her knees were cut, and she was in great distress. Her knees and hands were bleeding, and she also had a black eye. She could not get back into the house, as she did not have her key, and she was frightened to go to the door on her own as Jimmy was still inside. She could not leave the close mouth as it was about time for Jim's school bus to arrive. Sometime later Jim's school bus turned the corner and arrived at the close. As Jim stepped down from the school bus, and saw the state that his Mammy was in he got the fright of his life. "What happened ?" asked wee Jim, he was in shock; he asked over, and over again what had happened.

Edna, Cathie's neighbour and friend took them in and bathed and cleaned up Cathie's cuts and bruises, and made Cathie and Jim something to eat. "I think you should charge him" said Edna. "I will get the police to give him a warming" replied Cathie. Cathie and Edna went to the police station and asked them to come down with them and give Jimmy a warning, saying that she did not want to charge him, but she would like to get some clothes and belongings for Jim and herself out of the house. The police came down to the house with them, and Edna got her pram into which Cathie put articles of clothing for Jim and herself, as much as Edna's pram could carry. By this time it was getting dark again and the rain was starting. Half-way down the road Cathie told Edna, "he has had his last chance, never again, I'm not going back on no account am I going back". They arrived at Granda's close and bumped the pram up the stairs. It was very heavy. They chapped the door, and it was opened, "Not again ?" asked Granda. "Yes again" replied Cathie. "Come in, your usual room madam ? this is beginning to get like a hotel". "That's it this time Da, there is no way that I am going back to that man" she said.

Cathie and Jim felt safe down at Granda's home. Jim liked it down there with Jackie and all his old pals. Auntie May and Auntie Ellen still lived at home along with Margaret and Big John and wee Jackie. As Cathie and Jim still had their old room it was like old times; they felt very much at peace and very contented. Jim and Jackie could go down to the backcourt or up to the old farm land and have a great time playing with their pals, like before.

Cathie telephoned the school and explained to the headmistress, who was a nice old soul, the situation that Jim and she were in, and ask to arrange for the school bus to collect Jim at his Grandfathers home; this was arranged and Jim continued with his education.

After a few weeks Cathie got herself a job in "Brand & Mollison", the dry cleaners up in Cranston Hill which was handy for Jim's school. Cathie took a great interest in Jim's education, and made regular visits to the school to enquire about Jim's progress. The teacher was always glad to see her, and told Cathie that she only looked like a wee girl herself, and that she wished that other parents would take the same interest in their children. Jim still had to attend the speech and physiotherapy clinics for treatment, and still having to miss a lot of his schooling. Some days when the shop was quiet, Cathie's boss, Miss Paul, would let Cathie go away early at three o'clock to meet Jim at school and collect him before he went on the school bus to go home. The school bus attendant, also a Miss Dougherty, was an old friend of Cathie's. Cathie took Jim to visit another of her friends, Susie and her husband Jimmy, who lived with their five of a family in Dover Street. Young Jim loved it there, it was a happy house. The one room and kitchen house was in the close, and the door was never locked. Neighbours and friends just opened the main door and walked straight in, shouting, "It's me Susie, I'm just in to use your toilet", they used it and went straight out again. Someone would ask "Who was that ?" and Susie would reply, "I don't know !" They felt safe in their homes. The big long lobby was dark, as the light switch was at the other end. The long lobby had a big pulley hanging from the middle of the ceiling, which Susie used every day to hang up her washing when the weather was bad and it could not be hung up in the backcourt. Susie's husband, Uncle Jimmy worked very hard at an engineering factory, and also helped to run an athletic club. He trained the young runners, and was out a lot. They were a very loving couple, and every time he would go out , they would kiss each other; Jim would say to his Mammy that he liked it in their house as all the children could go into the room and play at pilots parashooting from their planes ; the children jumped from the wardrobe down to the bed in the room it was a wonder that they did not break the springs.

Money was very tight with, as in many homes, only one wage coming in. Susie, like many other mothers, found it very hard to make ends meet. She would say to one of her children, "Here is a shopping list, take it to the shop at the corner and get the messages, and tell the shop owner to put it on the slate, and I'll settle up with him at the end of the week". Lots of families had to do this to help them get through the week, as wages were not good. The grocer knew that he would always get the money from Susie at the end of the week when she got her wages from Jimmy. In fact he wished that all his customers were as good payers. He would feel sorry for some of his customers who would not, or could not pay him at the end of the week, and run up big bills. The grocer would then have a hard job trying to get the money that was owned to him. The customers would then get black-listed, and were told "Nae mere tick, until you pay up" as they entered the shop, and it was very enbarracing to the grocer and other customers in the shop. Some poor souls had no money to feed their families and had to go to a money lender to get themselves out of a hole, and they would charge them extortionate interest. The corner shop was also handy for getting pennies for the gar and electric meters.

There was a woman visitor who came to Susie's house, and everyone said that she was good at reading the cups. All the women would visit and sit round the table, and they would all have a cup of tea and something to eat. After the ladies had drunk their tea they turned their cups upside down onto the saucer and turn it around three times, and then they waited their turn to have their cup read. The Spaywife would then proceed to read the tea leaves in the cup and tell the women things like, "Oh, I see the leaves are good to you". She would say things like "I see a tall dark handsome man, and he is bringing you good tidings". Wee Nellie said that it was true, a big man with dark hair came to empty her gas meter, and Wee Nellie got five bob rebate. She told Cathie things like "Oh, Ah see a wee bird in the leaves and its to bring you a message from afar", and she continued "Ah see a £ sign, look, do you see it?" Cathie and the rest of the ladies around the table would say "Yes" just to please her, and she would carry on, "Aye, you're coming into money, hen. You're either gone'y win the pools, or your old mans gone'y snuff it, and your gone'y get his insurance money". She would bell Big Sadie, who she knew was dying for a man, "Your gone'y meet a tall dark handsome stranger with a view to romance".

Cathie and her pals would save up their money for weeks to go to see a right fortune teller, a Mrs. Bird, and she sat on a high chair, like a parrot on a perch. "God bless the mark, my God, she is like a bird on a perch right-enough; The women would walk up to Overnoughton, up the street, up the stairs, and knocked on the door, in great expectation. The would open and Mrs. Bird's wee friend would tell them to come and take a seat on the row of chairs that were lined up against the wall of the long lobby. They would sit down and await their turn to go into the room where Mrs Bird would tell their fortune. One by one they would enter the room, "Sorry, only yin at a time, hen, Ah' can'y see two o' you at wans. Ah"ll tell your fortune moo hen, would you like your palm read, or Ah can read the cards if you like and you can give the money tae wee Ina on the way oot. Noo sit doon, hen, and she proceeded to tell the fortune of each of the ladies. Jessie was first, and when she came out she said to the other woman, who were still waiting their turn. "She's awfy good, she told me things about my family that she could'nae possibly know", she told the other women, then Jessie said "Ah can'nae mind half o'what she told me, she goes very fast". The rest of the other woman said the same, still, it was a good night out for the women, and they all enjoyed themselves, and had a good laugh and a bag of chips to eat going down the road. "That was a better night out than those men o' oors would have standing in a pub, propping up the bar and arguing about horses and football", said Susie. "Fortune ! The old Bird is the only one that made a fortune", said Jessie as they went home.

Chapter Seven
ANOTHER CHANCE

Cathie and wee Jim settled very nicely into their room at Granda's home. Cathie was very happy in her job at the cleaners, and Jim at school. Cathie became very popular with the customers at the drycleaners where she worked. The customers regularly brought in their suits to be dry-cleaned and their shirts to be laundered, and there was also a bag-wash, where the customers put their dirty washing in a bag to get washed, to save them the time of going to the wash-house or the "steamie". Most of the mothers with big families took their washing to the Steamie. Once or twice a week they would get up very early in the morning and put all their washing into an old pram, with their soap-powder and scrubbing board. They got a stall which was allocated to them by the attendant. It was very hard work for the women, but they enjoyed themselves, as it got them out of the house, and away from their families for awhile. They also got a laugh, and it was a chance to catch up on all the local gossip. They would tell eachother things like: "poor Jeanie is to go into hospital... wuman's trouble", and old Mrs Craig said, "Did you hear, ma Katie is expecting again, that big swine that she's married to should go and take a run and jump, and I don't mean on the bed. Naw, he's done enough damage there already, that's six wains, she's got noo". The women liked to sing songs like "Dont fence me in" and someone shouted "your fenced in already". They had to hurry home to get their messages in and their housework done and the dinner on for the wains coming home from school, and their men from their work.

Cathie was a good listener, and the customers would come into the cleaners and stop to chat, or a "wee blether", and tell her of their problems with their families, and they money worries and also their health problems. Some poor souls were just lonely and wanted to talk to someone; and it helped to pass the time for Cathie, as it was a long day when the shop was quiet.

Miss Paul, the manageress of the shop was a real lady; very formal. She liked to be called Miss; very prim and proper. Cathie and she got on very well. Miss Paul would sit in the back shop at lunch-time and tell Cathie of her travels, especially her trip to Helsinki in Finland. She had also been on holiday to France and many other European countries. She took great joy in telling Cathie her travellers' tales. Cathie would say, I would love to be a tourist, but she could only dream.

Cathie was competent in the management of the shop, and she was asked to be deputy manager of the shop wile Miss Paul was on her holiday break. Male customers came into the shop to have their shirts laundered, their collars turned, and their suits cleaned. They would come back hard and stiff, (the collars, not the men). Some of the men asked Cathie if she would like to go out with them. The toffs would say, "Cathie how would you like to come out to the theatre, or go for a meal ?" and the others would ask her, "Cathie, hen, do you fancy a wee night oot way me to the flicks, or goin' to the jigging ?" Cathie always declined their invitations. "Oh, my God no, I've had enough of men", she would say. Now, she just lived for her wee son.

Jim was getting on a lot better at school. There was a great improvement in his work, especially his reading and spelling, which always gave him cause for concern. He was very self-conscious in the class if he was asked to stand up and read out a passage from a book, or a piece of his work; Jim did not like to look a fool in front of his schoolfriends, especially, Kathleen. Jim developed a system, he knew that each child in the class would be told by the teacher to read a paragraph of a book, and he would count the number of children that had to read before him, and then count the same number of paragraphs down the book, and rehearsed it to read out in front of the class. Sometimes it worked, but there were times when the teacher asked another child to read longer, and Jim would lose the place when it came to his turn to read. He thought, so much for that system, I will just have to do better at my reading, and he did. He did not like being taken out and punished, by getting the strap or belt across the hand from the teacher in front of the class. The school was staffed by all woman teachers and headmistress. Most of them, old spinsters, who did not like children very much. They all liked giving the strap. One day a girl was very rude to the teacher, the girl refused to take the strap for being impertinent. The teacher lost her temper and took the girl out in front of the class put the girl over her knee and spanked the girl on the bottom; and Jim along with most of the class could see her knickers. They could be quite cruel.

The highlight of the school year was the annual trip, for all the special schools, to Balloch Park. It was the only chance that some of the pupils got to leave the city. They got very excited about it. Buses decorated with streamers and balloons would arrive at the entrance of each special school in the city. The children and teachers would board the buses at the entrance of each school at nine, just as the school bell rang, and each child would be given a bag of sweets to eat on the journey. As the buses drove off the children began to sing, they hoped for good weather, but it was nearly always raining. As they left the city to drive through the countryside, the sight of a cow or sheep caused great excitement to some of the children, who had not seen the animal before. Once they arrived at Balloch Park they went with the teachers and their helpers to a great big marquee. They all lined up to receive the packed lunch, which consisted of an apple, a cake, sandwiches and a cold pie, also a bottle of milk or juice. They played games and had races, and watched a Punch & Judy show. Policemen were in attendance and two of them took Jim and a couple of others for a sail on Loch Lomond. It started to rain and it was soon time to return to Glasgow. It was the talking point for days and weeks to come for some of the children.

It was back to the more mundane things in the world of lessons in school, reading, sums. However the teacher gave them some work that would let them express their day at Balloch. The days that the children misbehaved in class, or produce very bad work, the teacher knew that they had not been trying, and their work was really untidy or dirty. Miss Doughtery took them out in front of the class and gave them the belt, or the strap. Cathie took a great interest in Jim's education, and made regular visits to the school to enquire about his progress.

Wee Jim and Cathie were very content living down in Granda's home and enjoyed the company of the other members of the family who were still living at home. They always went out on a Saturday night. Cathie would take Jim to the pictures or to visit friends, or others in the family who had got married and moved away: Or, Cathie said to Him, what picture would you like to go and see, and she would read out all the films that where showing that week in the various picture halls in the district; There was always two films showing in each cinema, a good American A film, which was the main feature, and a British B movie, which the people in Glasgow always thought was awful, because they thought that the films wee too English. It was a great nights entertainment, two films, a cartoon, and a newsreel, not forgetting the trailers, "For your future entertainment" and went on and on and on... showing trailers of bits of films that would be coming to the picture hall for weeks to come. They practically gave the plot way. The Hollywood musicals were very good, and Cathie and Jim enjoyed seeing films like "Singing in the rain" with Gene Kelly, "Annie get your gun" and "Oklahoma". They had to queue for half an hour, or sometimes up to an hour, in the cold and rain to get in to see the picture. Jim would get cold and fed-up and tired, and say to his Mammy "I want to go home, I'm tired, or, I'm cold and hungry, come on let's just go home". Just then the commitioner would come out and say, "come on room for some more, then more seats inside, and Cathie and Jim would get in, and after a long wait they had missed the start of the first film. The auditorium was very dark and the usherette shawn a torch down the aisle to let the patrons find their seats, when she found a row with empty seats, the usherette would shine her torch along the row, and shout at the people sitting in the seats, "come on, move along, shub up, and make room for more in the row" in her sargent-magors voice; She liked to shine her torch on the couples winching in the backrow;

Cathie and Jim frequently enjoyed the cinema. It was a continuous programme, and people would be coming and going all through the films, and Jim and Cathie, and the other patrons had to move their heads from side to side to try to see the screen, and people would go out to buy ice-cream and sweets. Jim would complain to Cathie, and say "I cant see a thing Mammy, that man in front of me has a big head" or, "the woman in front of me has a hat that is to big for her head, but then, maybe she has got a big head". Cathie replied, "and you have got a big mouth, shut-up and watch the picture". The film came round to the part that they had come in at, and Cathie said, "Its time to go home", and Jim would say "let's stay a wee while longer to see another wee bit of the film". Cathie agreed, then after Jim had seen that bit, he wanted to see another wee bit. "Right; that's it, home" said Cathie, and Jim left the film with some reluctance. But he knew that if Auntie Ellen had not seen the picture, that she would take Jackie and him to see it again. Cathie and Jim left the picture hall, and as usual the rain had started, it was coming down in buckets, "O' God, look at the rain and we have got nothing to cover our heads". Normally Jim wore his brown school cap, but only liked to wear it to school, and Cathie normally had a head-scarf in her bag, but it had been a lovely dry evening when they left home. They made their way to the tramcar stop, and being a Saturday, there was a long queue and a couple of tramcars passed by without stopping, as they were jam-packed with passengers. "We'll never get home at this rate" said Cathie. "I'm tried, cold and fed-up" said Jim. A tramcar eventually stopped and they managed to get on, just. "Standing room only" cried the big fat conductress. The "Old Firm" Celtic and Rangers were playing a local derby at Parkhead, the result had been a draw, so there was not the same amount of fighting, and both sets of supporters were coming on and getting off at various pubs on route, along with people from the picture halls along the route of the tramcar journey. Everyone was in party mood, the Celtic fans singing "Sure, its a grand old team to play for", and the Rangers fans singing "Follow, follow, we will follow Rangers". As the tramcar continued on its journey along Dumbarton Road, a party atmosphere prevailed, with more party songs, and the drink was flowing from the carry-outs. "Open a screw-top" said one fan, "want a wee hauf?" said another, "Gees a wee swally" asked another, to this big bloke, "away" and buy your ain "F"ing drink" was the reply. "That's no language to use in front of children and ladies" shouted this wee wuman. "Away and boil your heid, and put a sock in it you greetin' face auld bag". "That's nae yae tae talk tae a wuman"; "Oh' shut your face Mrs. gees another swig o' yur screw-tap big man", said the drunk fan. A fight broke out between opposing fans, and at this stage the big breasted conductress, who had been up on the top deck collecting fares, came hurrying down the stairs, with her ticket machine bobbing up and down on her large chest, appeared on the scene, she interrupted the troublemakers, shouting at the top of her voice "Ah've been up the stairs, collecting fares and Ah heard O' the commotion doon the stairs , and" she added, "'Come oon, get aff A' yuse trouble makers". At this stage a wee man with a bad leg and a checked bunnit came on the car with a fish supper in his hand at Whiteinch Cross, right between the fighting fans. The wee man had a wee drink in him, and asked, "Anybody want a chip?" At this stage a fan made a dive for a chip, and the wee mans fish supper went flying through the air. "That's ma tea" said the wee man "Ah'm starving". At this someone shouted "never mind wee man, you could be doing with losing some weight"; and everyone burst out laughing. "That's a shame" said this woman and had whip-round to buy the wee man another fish supper. Now, two policemen came on and order was restored. The tramcar continued on along Dumbarton Road, stopping at every stop to let passengers on and off. Cathie and Jim were very relieved when they reached their destination; After they had crossed the road to the pavement they could smell the lovely smell of chips coming from the fish and chip shop. It was owned by Italians, and everyone in Glasgow knew that they made the best fish suppers. The commotion on the tramcar with the wee man's fish and chips along with the aroma coming from the fish and chip shop, put them in the mood for chips. They went in and waited in the queue to be served. As usual, the chips were not ready, and the woman behind the counter said, "They will no be long, hen" to Cathie, and Jim knew what that meant – they could be in the shop for ages, he had counted nine customers to be served before them. Once the chips were ready, the girl serving from behind the counter asked for their order again. Cathie said "two bags of chips, Oh' and a bottle of Tizer please". The queue moved along, and Jim said, "Oh' good we're getting nearer, and I'm busting for the bathroom". The girl behind the counter asked Cathie to repeat her order. At last with their chips and Tizer they made their way home and it was still raining, but chips taste better in a wet bag with newspapers and the vinegar oozing out. They made their way to the house, and when they got in Granda was in the livingroom listening to the wireless, and writing out his racing lines from the tips that he got from the newspapers. Margaret and Big John were in their room listening to the new records that they had bought that day, and Little Jackie was in his bed fast asleep. It was a happy time.

The next day, being a Sunday they all got up early, except Big John, who liked a long lie-in, and Granda, who spent all day on a Sunday in bed reading the Sunday papers. The rest of the family got up and ready with their Sunday best on, and went to Mass. If they were going to receive Holy Communion, they did not have breakfast, as they had to fast from mid-night the night before. Sometimes they got a tramcar to the chapel, if it was raining, or if they were late. They arrived at the chapel and sat in the back row, as Jackie tended to be noisy, and some of the older priests tended to go on preaching for a long time, and repeating themselves, thought Margaret. Jackie ran away from Margaret and before the passkeeper could catch him he had ran up onto the high alter as the priest was offering up the Blessed Sacrament for Holy Communion. The woman sitting next to Margaret could not contain herself, as she started laughing, and had to put a hankie in her mouth to deaden the sound of her laughter. When Jim was younger he thought that the confessional box was Gods bathroom, and always wanted in for a pee; and he told Jackie this, and he started shouting at the pitch of his voice that he wanted to go into Gods bathroom for a "wee wee", and Margaret had to take him outside.

Jimmy was always coming down to ask Cathie for a reconciliation. He was desperate to get Cathie to go back with him. "I've changed, I'm a changed man,, no more drinking for me, no more drinking with my mates after work. I'll come straight home with my wages. Things will be different this time". He kept repeating. He continued "I miss you and Jim very much, please come back". Like lots of other women, Cathie had heard it all before. However she decided to give him the benefit of the dout, and she agreed to return to him.

The following day Cathie packed her belongings and returned to live with Jimmy, and gave him another (one last) chance; "Will I come down and help you up the road with your belongings ?" he asked her. "No, I will come on my own", she told him. When she arrived she found that he had the house looking like a new pin and a nice meal all prepared ready to serve. They stayed on their own that first night back together, and probably their third child was conceived then; The following day Jim arrived, and they were a united family again.

Cathie had to telephone the school again, to have the school bus collect Jim at his own home again. When Jim boarded the school bus the following day the children on board were asking awkward questions, like "why are you moving back from one house to another and then back again ?"

The neighbours were very pleased to see them back again, the ones that they got on with. Jim was glad to see old Mr. Hay and all his old pals again. After a couple of days it was like he had never been away. He had a lot of catching up to do;

At school, Jim was in the first Holy Communion class, and the children were preparing to receive the Blessed Sacrament for the first time, and also their first confession. They were also progressing with their normal school work, and Jim had a keen interest in the subjects of geography and history. He liked to read of the Scottish Kings and Queens, and of different countries and their capitals and their inhabitants. As it was the first Holy Communion class, the priest from the local chapel, which was Saint Patrick's, would come to the class a couple of times a week to give instruction on Bible history and catechism. One day the class walked down from St. Martin's to the church of St. Patrick's for a rehearsal, and to make their first confession. The teacher made the children walk in a straight line, like animals going into the ark; "No talking, in a straight line" said the teacher. It was the same when they went for swimming lessons to Cranstonhill baths.

Jim was extremely excited when the day that he was to make his First Holy Communion had finally arrived. His nervous tension had built up to fever pitch. Cathie had to give him one of his phenabarbatone pills to calm him down. The night before she had him bathed and into bed early, although it took him ages to get to sleep, it was a very long night as he tossed and turned in bed, thinking about the next day, and listening for the nice, who eventually came out to play, until Tibby the cat caught one. The morning finally arrived and Cathie shouted to waken him. Jim felt as if he had just fallen to sleep, and wanted to turnover, and go back to sleep. "Come on, up you get Jim", shouted Cathie, yet again. Jim finally had to get up. "I'm tired and fed-up" said Jim. "Well, you will just have to be", replied Cathie. "This is the happiest day of your life" she continued. "You could have fooled me", thought Jim, if God meant me to happy He would have given me a long lay-in". Once he was up and washed,

Jim said, "I'm hungry, can I have something to eat?" "No" was the reply from his Mammy "Your going to make your First Holy Communion, and you can't eat anything after Midnight on the previous night. He got ready for the big occasion, new suit, new shoes, and shirt and tie, socks and underwear. He looked the part; "All ready, do you need to go to the toilet?" asked Cathie. "I may as well go again", and Jim went again, as he was always going to the toilet at the last minute as they were in a hurry to leave the house. "For goodness sake hurry-up, we're going to be late", said Cathie, as they left to get the tramcar to Saint Patrick's Church in Anderston. It was a Thursday, and all the other children and their mothers and some of the fathers were in the pews, most of the fathers could not get time off from work; Cathie, and the rest of the parents sat in the centre of the church, the rest of the congregation at the back. Pride of place for the first communicians was at the front of the church.

Jim was feeling very shaky as he sat waiting for the Mass to begin, "Whit's up wae you?" asked the boy sitting next to Jim. "Nothing", was Jim's reply. "Well stop shaking then" said the boy, and this made Jim worse. Jim looked over to where the girls were sitting, and they all looked lovely in their white dresses and veils, especially, Kathleen, the girl he liked in the school. Canon Boland, a big figure of a man, came out with the alter boys to celebrate the Mass. The children said their prayers and sang the hymns which they had been learning for months in the class at the school. The highlight of the Mass was when the children went up to the alter rails in pairs, a boy from one side of church and a girl from the other, Jim hoping that he would get Kathleen to walk up to the alter with. They knelt at the alter rails and received the Blessed Sarcament, and returned to their seats. The children knew that Our Lord and Our Blessed Lady were looking after them, and that they had received the body and blood of Our Lord Jesus Christ. After the Mass the Canon congratulated them, and wished them a happy and holy life, and not to forget to attend Mass and perform their duties as they grew older. The children left the church to be congratulated by their mothers and then had to return to St. Martin's school, where a large breakfast was waiting for them in the dining hall. It consisted of ham, egg and sausages with rolls and cups of tea. The children were starving and got "stuck-in" to the meal. "What did you think of the host ?" asked Wee Pat. "I didn't taste it, I just swallowed it like the teacher told me", Jim replied. The rest of the day was spent in the school, but the children did not get any work to do. The day had been a holy one.

When Jim returned home from school on the school-bus, his Auntie May, who was his Godmother was waiting at the house for him, she had got away from her work early to take Jim down to the photographers in Partick to have his picture taken in his First Communion suit, and then took him home again as Cathie was not feeling very well, and she had to be in for Jimmy's tea. In the photographic studio, Jim had to stand very still for what seemed a very long time to him, as the photographer got him to stand in the right position, and stand very still, as Jim said to himself, "Oh' for goodness sake get on with it"; He was dying to get home and get out of his clothes and get on his old clothes and get out to play with his pals.

Chapter Eight
ANOTHER FALL & A HOLIDAY

Cathie suspected that she might be pregnant again, and she was not very pleased. The football season had started, and Jimmy was beginning to fall by the wayside, as they say, with his drinking. She made an appointment to go to the doctor's surgery to have a pregnancy test, which proved positive. She worried about having two children in the wee single-end. She put off telling Jimmy for a couple of days, not that he minded, Cathie was just not in the mood for telling him, and when she did he was very pleased, and they hoped for a girl this time.

They went to the housing department of the Glasgow Corporation and asked to be considered for a larger house, as they had their names on their waiting list for some years. They got told that there was a long waiting list, and that it would be years before they could be considered for rehousing. They went to Dr. Gallagher and explained the situation to him, and he gave them a medical certificate regarding Jim's condition. It did not help them to be re-housed, and they had to stay in the single-end for the time being.

Two months later Margaret also discovered that she too was expecting a baby, and this brought the two sisters, although Margaret was twelve years younger than Cathie, closer. Together they went to the antenatal clinic. They also went to the shops to buy baby clothes. They also bought wool, as Cathie was a good knitter, and she started to knit two shawls. As it would take her quite a long time to knit two she started to work on them early on in their pregnancies. She knitted other things, like cardigans. Margaret said to her, "I don't know who you do it, I wouldn't have the patience"; May was good at knitting socks, and started to work on bootees for the two new arrivals. They both put money down on new prams, but did not get them until after the babies were born, as they thought that it was bad luck to have the prams in the house before the children were born. Both had trouble free pregnancies, and Cathie's baby was born first. It was another boy, they had hoped for a girl this time, but Cathie and Jimmy were both pleased that the baby was alright this time, and Cathie had no trouble during the birth. They both agreed to call the baby Thomas, after Cathie's brother, and Tommy's wife, Mary was asked to be the Godmother. A week or two after the baby was born, Thomas was taken by Mary up to St. Ninian's church to get christened, as it was considered bad not to get the baby christened as soon as possible incase anything should happen to the baby. The baby was wrapped in Jim's christening shawl, it was used by each new baby born into the family. Mary took the baby to the chapel, in her arms she had the baby and the christening piece. This piece was a paper bag in which was a piece of cake or biscuit, and a silver coin for luck, and Mary gave it to the first female that she met on her way to the chapel. If the baby had been female, then the christening piece would go to a male. Thomas was a small baby, but very healthy with lovely fair hair, almost white, the women loved it, and he was a very good sleeper, not like his older brother, Jim. Some days he would sleep to near lunch time. Two months later Margaret gave birth to her baby, it too was another boy, and she and Big John decided to name him Francis after the other brother Frank. The baby was to be called Frankie. He was a very large baby unlike Jackie, who was very small and dark. Frankie was large and blond. Margaret asked her sister Ellen to be the Godmother, she was as pleased as punch, and took her roll very seriously.

Jimmy was still working as a slater and plasterer, and was working up on a steeple of a church in Linlithgow, then he fell off again, twice this has happened, "Is God trying to tell him something ?" Cathie wondered; Another chapel roof. The housekeeper from the chapel house found him laying on the ground in a pool of blood, and he was unconscious. She rushedto get the priest, and they attended to him until the ambulance arrived to take him to the hospital in Edinburg. Jimmy was rushed to the Royal Infirmary, where they discovered that he had multiple injuries, consisting of broken limbs: two broken arms, two broken legs and head and facial injuries. He was a very ill man. When he did not arrive home for his tea Cathie thought the obvious, "That swine has gone to get drunk again". Then she thought, "It's the middle of the week, and he has no money for drink, and he did not bother with the horse racing. He must have met someone who had a win and they've taken him for a pint or two... That's another ruined meal", Cathie said to herself, as she sat looking at the clock, and getting the boys ready for their bed. Just then there was a knock on the door. It was the police, who had received a telephone call from the Royal Infirmary asking them to inform Cathie of what had happened to Jimmy, and it was the same two policemen who had been the last time Jimmy had started his nonsense. "How's that man of yours been behaving himself ?" they asked Cathie. "Oh' you know the same as usual" she replied. "Well, he'll not be misbehaving himself for a long time", and they told her about his injuries. Cathie went to her bed and the next morning she got up early and got the boys ready and fed, and took them down on the tramcar to their Granda's house. As she got to the door, it was opened as Margaret heard the sound of them coming up the stair. The first thing that was asked, was : "Has that man been causing you trouble again ?" Cathie told them what had happened, her mind was in turmoil, she did not know what to do; "Leave the children with us, and you can go to Edinburgh yourself, and find out what happened"; Cathie made her way by tramcar up to the station and bought a day return ticket to Edinburgh. After she arrived at Waverley station she got a taxi to the Royal Infirmary. After she arrived at the ward, she went to see the doctor, who informed her of the extent of Jimmy's injuries. When she went into the ward and saw the state that Jimmy was in, she said to him, "Oh' my God what has happened to you ? You're in some state". He replied, "I fell". He was laying in bed with very bad head, face and limb injuries, and the doctor was worried as to the extent of his head injury, and he would need bone-grafts on his legs.

He was hospitalized for a long time, and Cathie faithfully made the train trip to the Capital two or three times a week to visit Jimmy, sometimes taking one or both of the boys with her on her visits. Jim enjoyed the train trip to Edinburgh, and seeing the Castle, he was really interested in his father's injuries. After sometime, Jimmy was transferred to a rehabilitation hospital in Bridge of Weir. Jim loved going out there, not so much to see his Daddy, but he loved the bus ride out into the country and the lovely salad rolls that you got with the juice in the hospital cafeteria. It was a good day out for Jim in the summer, but was a terrible ordeal in the winter when the weather was bad. Cathie and Jim standing at the bus stop in the wind and rain; although they were dressed for the weather with their raincoats and fishermans' hats.

Sometimes Jimmy's sister Vea and her husband Bill visited the hospital to see Jimmy, and would invite Cathie and Jim to their home for tea. They stayed in the house that had been the home of Jimmy's parents. Jimmy's older brother, Jack was good at playing the organ, and Jim liked to have a go. They also had an old gramophone, with a wind-up handle, and their parents old 78r.p.m. records to play on it. Jim and his cousin, Davina were going through the old records one Sunday, and found one that had been re-released, and was in the charts. "Fancy that being in beside all this old rubbish", said Jim. Davina put the record on and they played it over and over, and as the speed of the turntable slowed down, they had to turn the handle fast to speed the record turn-table up again to hear the recording at the right speed. They had a nice dog that Jim liked to take out for a walk on the lead, but one day the dog turned on Jim and bit him. Before that, Jim always said that he would like a dog, but that experience put him off dogs for years. Jimmy's older brother, Uncle Jack liked to play the organ, and was quite good. He liked classical music, and attended concerts in the St. Andrew's Halls, Glasgow. One Saturday evening, he took young Jim to a concert, but Jim was not to impressed, although he liked some of the music, he preferred the music that was in the record charts. However, Jim liked it when the concert was finished, and Uncle Jack took him to a cafe for hot chocolate drink on the way home. When they got home to Jim's home, Uncle Jack asked Jim how he enjoyed the concert. Jim replied, "Very much", as he did not want to up-set his Uncle Jack, as it was very good of him to take Jim.

When Jimmy returned home from hospital, he could walk with the aid of two walking sticks, and then one. He contacted a solicitor to apply for compensation, and after a lot of negotiation, he received the sum of £3,000 compensation. A fortune in 1952. What a windfall – a great way to keep Cathie and the children for good, Jimmy thought to himself, and started to make plans. He thought about buying a "Shooting Break", but he could not drive. Then he thought about asking Big John to drive it, "Not a good idea" said Cathie. Jimmy had not many good ideas. Cathie said to him, "look Jimmy, we will sit down and make plans that are to benefit the family, you, me, and the boys". This they did, and they began to make their plans to put the money to good use. "Will you reconsider opening a bank account in Jim and Thomas's names", asked Cathie. Jimmy replied, "I'll think about it", but he never did.

Television, a new media, had just arrived and the B.B.C. had begun testing transmissions of their programmes to Central Scotland from the transmitter at Kirk O' Shotts. To coincide with the event, an exhibition was held in the St. Andrew's Halls in Kent Road. Jim was fascinated by the new media, a radio with pictures, as Jim called it. A wonderful new invention by a fellow Scot, John Logie Baird. The family were fascinated as they walk around the darkened hall looking at the 9 inch and 12 inch screen models. There were table models, and console sets that had doors on them, to keep the screens clean, when not in use. Jimmy said to Cathie "Oh' come on and we will buy one", and wee Jim said, "Yes get one, a wireless in the house with pictures would be just great". Cathie replied, "Just wait a minute, there are more important things that we need for the house before a television". They walked through a door into a room which had been made into a studio. It had all the equipment that was used to produce programmes, a control room, cameras and microphones. From there they proceeded into the main hall, were an audience participation programme was going out on the air. It consisted of two artists' drawing the faces of famous people, whose names the audience called out. Jim said to his parents that he did not recognise some of the faces that they had drawn. He could perceive that the new media would be a great success. On the way home, and all that week, Cathie and Jimmy talked of the pross and cons of buying a television set, and decided to put the idea on hold for time being, much to Jim's disappointment.

Cathie and Jimmy decided that a really good holiday would be their first priority. They thought that a holiday would revitalise thier lives, and give them and the two boys, Jim and Thomas, a new start. They took the boys down to Byers Road, to a travel agency. They looked through the holiday brochures, but did not fancy going to the Continent. They noticed a brochure for Butlin's Holiday Camps, owned by Billy Butlin. They liked the look of the camp in Mosney, near Dublin, the Capital

City of The Irish Republic. They booked up for two weeks holiday at the camp, and decided to spend an additional week in Dublin. They went out and bought a big trunk to pack all the new holiday clothes that they had bought to wear on the holiday. Cathie bought new dresses, shoes skirts and blouses. Jimmy bought a new suit, shoes and casual clothes, and a bicky-bow tie, to look the part of a real gentleman; and of course, the boys got new clothes too. The trunk was sent on ahead, and was there when they arrived. Cathie was worried sick that it might get lost en-route.

It was the day of their departure, and the taxi arrived to take them down to the Broomilaw to get the ship and said to Dublin. They had always been used to travelling steerage on their past holidays to Ireland, but, not this time. They travelled in style; and had booked a cabin. "Oh' the luxury of it" thought Cathie. They arrived at the docks and took their turn in the queue. They walked up the gangway onto the deck of the ship, and then were taken to be shown their cabin. Once they had settled in, the funnel blew and to the delight of the boys, "anchors away" and the ship set sail down the River Clyde, and out into the Irish Sea. Jim looked trough the port-hole on the wall of the cabin , and all that he could see was water, water, "that's all that I can see" he told his parents. Just then another ship passed going in the other direction. The family went for a meal, and then they went back to their comfortable cabin and settled down for a good night's sleep. "This beats sailing steerage anytime", said Jimmy, and Cathie and Jim agreed. They felt really refreshed after their wash, and went to have a nice big breakfast of ham, egg, sausage and tea and toast. The ship sailed up the River Liffey and docked at Dublin. Everyone was very excited. As they had to walk down the very long, very steep gangway, the boys were frightened, and Jim was relieved when he reached the bottom. They went straight into the customs shed and passed through with no bother. Out into the Dublin street, the weather was dull, with a slight drizzle of rain. On the road, by the side of the pavement stood a horse and carriage for hire. The family got in and asked the drive if he could take them to lodgings.

Jim notice a large pile of manure on the street under the horse and shouted, "Oh, jobbies", and he continued, "there is a large pile of jobbies under that horse". "Be quiet" said Cathie, and continued "you are on holiday to enjoy yourself, and if you don't be quiet and behave yourself, then you wont enjoy yourself". Jim got the message and kept quiet. Cathie and Jimmy and the two boys climbed into the carriage, and the driver put the big trunk onto the back. The family had not booked accommodation for their stay in Dublin, so they asked the carriage driver if he knew of bed and breakfast accommodation in the city. The carriage driver, who was called Pat and was a very friendly man. He said that he knew a boarding house that had a room to let, and that the landlady was a good friend of his wife. She liked children, and was not too expensive. "Good, that sounds ideal" said Cathie. "Please take us there" asked Jimmy, and the horse and carriage drove off. On the way to the boarding house they had a chance to see some of the sights of Dublin. After a drive of about twenty minutes, or half-an-hour (they enjoyed the ride so much that the did not really notice the time). They arrived at their destination. The boarding house looked alright from the outside. The carriage driver put on the breaks and got down from the carriage. He went up the steps to the boarding house and chapped on the door, which was opened by a short middle-aged woman with white hair. She was dressed all in black. Pat, the carriage driver spoke to her for a minute, and then beckoned to the family to come up and meet . Mrs. O'Kane, who said that she had a nice room, with two double beds that would be ideal for their stay. They agreed the terms of the let and Jimmy and the driver went down to the carriage to get the trunk, while Cathie and the boys made their way up the stairs with Mrs. O'Kane to be shown their room. It was clean and bright, but had no wash-hand basin, instead there was a large bowl with a jug of cold water for washing hands and face. Cathie, thought to herself, its only for five days, we'll manage; Just then Jim noticed a large chamber pot under one of the beds and shouted, "There's a big pot, he actually said "chanty" under the bed. Mrs O'Kane laughed, and said "breakfast at nine", and made her way out of the room.

They had a rest and then a wash and put on a change of clothes. Then they went out to find somewhere to have a meal and also to explore the City of Dublin, which has many interesting places to visit and sights to see. By day Cathie and Jimmy took Jim and Thomas, who had just begun to walk, and smart on his feet, to visit the lovely zoo and parks. One day they strolled along O'Connel Street, they came to the bottom of Nelson's Column in the centre of the street, and decided to enter the door and walk up the steps all the way to the top, which was really a tiring tast. As they walked up the stairs Jimmy carried Thomas. Jim found the strain of walking up all the stairs very hard-going and was very glad when they finally reached the top, until he looked down to see the panoramic view, to discover that he did not have a head for heights. He was absolutely terrified, stood with his back against the wall, and would not go near the railing, which was closed in at the top with wire netting to stop people jumping off to their deaths. "Let's go down the stairs" said Cathie, "we have been up here long enough"; "You can say hat again" replied Jim, who did not relish the though of having to walk down all those steps again to get to the bottom. He was glad when he finally arrived there.

Cathie and Jimmy liked to go round all the lovely shops in Dublin, as goods in the shops were inexpensive compared to the United Kingdom. They bought presents to take home and also a new camera. As the boys got a little tired of going around the shops Cathie said that it would be a good idea to take them on a day trip on the train to Bray for the day to let them play on the beach and get some good sea air. The boys enjoyed their trip along the coast on the train, and when the arrived in the town they went to a shop and bought buckets and spades to make sand castles. They also enjoyed taking off their shoes and socks and going for a paddle in the sea. After a couple of hours on the beach they all began to feel a bit hungry, "Lets go and find somewhere to eat" said Cathie. "I could go a pint", said Jimmy. "Never mind a pint, we'll find a cafe or restaurant and get a nice fish tea first" Cathie replied. This they did and got the train back to Dublin. There stay in Dublin was soon over and they had to pack their trunk and say Good-bye to Mrs. O'Kane. They told her how well that they had enjoyed there stay in Dublin, and thanked her as she had made them really lovely big breakfasts during their stay. Cathie and Jimmy and the boys got a carriage to take them and their trunk to the station to get the train to the destination of the second part of their holiday, which was Butlin's Holiday Camp along the coast at Mosney.

As Cathie, Jimmy and the boys arrived at the gates of the holiday camp all their faces lit up with happiness. The flags of many nations flew from the flag poles, the Red Coats, who helped and entertained in the camp were there to meet them, and they could hear the sound of all the latest music coming from the loudspeaker from the camp radio station. It was a very cheery atmosphere as the little train took them and their luggage past the swimming pool, the boating pond, and the skating ring to the reseption block, were they received the keys to their chalet and a time-table of meal-times and all the events and entertainment that was on offer in the camp. They, along with the other new arrivals, who had arrived on the same train were taken to find their chalets, which would be their home for the next two weeks. The chalets were in nice neat rows and brightly painted in different colours. They walked along the path, Jimmy, with the key swinging in one hand and his walking stick in the other. They preceded along the row until they found their number. Jimmy put the key in the lock and opened the door. Cathie's face lit up, as she walked in and sat down on the edge of the bed and said, "I think we are going to have a very good time here". The chalet had a main door in the middle of the wall with a window on each side and there was a double and a single bed and a cot for Thomas. The chalet also had a wash-hand basin with running hot and cold water which was appreciated after the bowl and jug in the boarding house in Dublin. Cathie began to unpack the big trunk again, as she said, "I hope the weather stays good, I've packed a lot of summer clothes, shorts and tee-shirts for the boys, and summer dresses for myself". Jim had also brought his denims, checked cowboy shirt, baseball boots and cap, which he felt good in; Jimmy went with Thomas to find out where the toilets and bathrooms were, and found them just across the other side of the path along with a wash-house. When he got back he told Cathie, she said, "That is a God-send, I've got things that I want to wash", and she went over to wash some clothes that had got dirty in Dublin. Then she put a rope across the front of the chalet to use as a washing line during their stay as the boys were always getting dirty, and needed clean clothes.

By this time they were feeling hungry, and as they had booked up for full board, three meals per day, it was time for them to go and look for the dining room. They eventually fond it, and it was just like a large works canteen. However it had waitress service, the food was good, and there was plenty of it, which was just as well, as they were all good eaters, (although you would'nt think it to look at Cathie, as she was very thin). Her mother used to say "I don't know where she puts all the food that she eats". Jimmy and Jim also had good appetites, in fact Jim did not know when to stop eating, but like his mother never got fat. Thomas ate in the baby dining room in the nursery, and the Red Coats looked after the children to let their parents go out on their own. Cathie and Jimmy went out of the camp on tours to the Guinnes Brewery and the Zoo in Dublin. They also visited the Hill of Tara, where they say that Saint Patrick vanished the snakes from Ireland, and with their new camera took pictures. Cathie also told Jim about the caves that they had visited there, and of the old woman, who was nearly blind, but took them down into the caves and with the light of a candle explained to them what the drawings on the walls meant.

Jim joined the Butlin's Beaver Club, and had the run of the camp. He went to all the club activities, and took part in some of the competitions, although he was hopeless at everything that he tried and never won anything, he liked the fun of taking part. He entered the best looking boy in the camp, and must have come in last. He had the nerve to enter the talent contest in the camp ballroom, and had the check to go on the stage and sing his song, "Roll a silver dollar" through the microphone, and he was so nervous that the microphone was shaking from side to side, and so was Jim. Cathie and Jimmy got the shock of their lives when the saw Jim on the film of camp events singing, or trying to. There were always contests going on in the holiday camp, Knobbly Knees, Glamorous Granny, Miss Butlin's and Bonnie Baby. Cathie did not enter Thomas, although she though that he had a good chance of winning. Cathie said that she did not believe in those kind of contests, she thought that all babies were beautiful. One day Thomas went missing from outside the chalet, and Cathie and Jimmy were very concerned as to his whereabouts, and a search party was sent out to look for him. He was found a short time later playing in the bathrooms, playing with his fathers walking stick in the toilet pan. Everyone was so relieved when he was found safe, and when he wondered off again they knew where to find him.

Jim enjoyed hiring a bicycle every day, if he was not going anywhere outside the camp, and would ride around for hours on end. Cathie did not worry about him, she knew that the exercise would do him good. He rode around all the shops, and the pubs and cafes, and to the camp radio station, to ask to have a record request played, and he would also ride down to the camp chapel, where they would have Mass on a Sunday.

One day Cathie and Jimmy invited a Belfast couple, a husband and wife, who they had met in Dublin back to the camp for the day and arranged to meet them as they came off the train at the main entrance. They took them on the camp train around the camp to show them all the attractions, and passed Jim, who was in a boat sailing in the boating pond. He gave them a wave with his hand and nearly fell in the pond. After that, he came off the boat and went to the skating rink to have a go at roller skating, and even with the help of a Red Coat, he could not stand on them.

When Jimmy saw Jim on the skates he had a daft idea, but Jimmy though that it was good at the time, of getting Jim to climb up onto the roof of the office where the skating rink attendant kept the skates to have his photograph taken with a large statue of a clown, standing on one hand.

Cathie and Jimmy took their friends to the swimming pool to watch the beauty contest and swimming events, and then they went for lunch. Cathie and Jimmy went to the camp restaurant, and their friends went to the visitors restaurant. After they had their meal they all met up again to go for a walk down to the beach, and then the men went to the bar for a pint, and the women went round the camp shops. Then Cathie met Jim and they went for a ride on the bicycles and they got a good photograph taken together. In the evening they took their friends to the theatre and to the ballroom for a drink before they left.

The children of the campers always came into the ballroom after the show in the theatre had finished. It was always a very entertaining show that they put on, with good turns. Singer and dancers and speciality acts. However, it was the same program every week, and the second week became a bit boring for Jim, who found other things to do, like go out on camp trips to Dublin Zoo, which he must have visited about three times. "It must be one of the most loveliest and best zoos in the world" he said to his parents.

The time in the ballroom had passed very quickly, and Cathie and Jimmy's visitors had to go home. As Cathie and Jimmy walked them to the main entrance of the camp they saw the last train back to Dublin leave. "What are we going to do now ?" asked the couple. "Well, there's only one thing for it" said Cathie, "We'll have to put you up for the night in our chalet" "How will you manage that ?" asked the couple, Peggy and Joe. "We'll just have to sneak you in. Thomas can sleep in our bed and Jim can sleep in the cot, and you will have to sleep in Jim's single bed". So the sneaked them back to their chalet, and without anyone noticing, and they all had a good nights sleep.

They got the first roll of film from the camera developed, and Cathie was very pleased with the results. She liked the photo of Jim and herself on the bicycle, and the photographs of Thomas, with his nice white hair. The second week at Butlin's flew in and it was time to get packed-up for the journey home. "It's been a great three weeks holiday, just great to get away from all that housework. Oh' the thought of going back to all that washing and ironing, going for message and cooking", said Cathie. "Ah' well its got to be done" she continued. They caught the train back to Dublin, and Jimmy said on the train "It has been a great and very pleasant three weeks". They got off the train in time to take a taxi to the docks to get the ship just in time to sail back to Glasgow, but they had a cabin booked and were sure to get a bed for the night, and a sleep. The next morning they had arrived back in Glasgow, and got off the ship feeling quite fresh and got a taxi home. When they arrived home Cathie opened the window to air the house, as it smelled a big fusty with being closed up for three weeks

The big trunk arrived back and Cathie got it opened. She got all the presents out, which they would take down to give to their family and friends, and then there was all the dirty washing !" I will have to get the boiler fired-up in the wash-house first thing on Monday morning to get this big washing done. I hope that the weather stays dry, and I can get it hung out on the line to dry. I'll need to go to the corner shop to get food in and something for the visitors". As Jimmy's sister and brother-in-law would be up to see how they got on during the holiday.

On the Sunday afternoon Cathie, Jimmy and the boys went down on the Number One tramcar to see Granda, May, Ellen, Margaret, Big John and Jackie to give them their presents from Ireland and show them the photographs of their holiday. Also, to hear also what had been happening at home whilst they were away. They talked for hours, Cathie and Jimmy telling them all about the great time that they had. The members of the family were very pleased with their presents. Ellen said, "I love these earrings, I will wear them to the dancing tomorrow night, up at the Playhouse". Ellen just loved the dancing, and she would go every night of the week, and afternoon too, if she had the money, but she took ill and had to give up work and go on the sick. She looked after the house while May was at work, still working in Carlaw's the Printers and Granda was still collecting lines for Magandy the bookie. Jim went down to the back to give wee Jackie his present, play with their pals, and tell them all about his holiday in their wee den that they had made of old tea chests and branches and big lengths of cardboard that they had found. The other children were not very interested in Jim's holiday, and must played on , and tried to improve the construction of their den. Sometime later Uncle Frank came to visit, and he had brought Eleanor, they had also been on holiday to Ireland, Donegal in fact. So when Eleanor came down to the back-court to play, Jim was very pleased to see her as they had a lot to talk about. Jim called out to her as soon as she saw her, "Hi, Eleanor come and tell me all about your holiday and I'll tell you all about mine".

As the children were playing out in the back-court the adults were talking about getting new homes. Cathie and Jimmy said that they would like a bigger house with an inside toilet, or a bathroom, and Margaret and Big John said that they had often talked about that and would love to move to a home of their own, more so now that they had two boys, Jackie and Frankie. They, too, like Cathie and Jimmy, had their name on Glasgow Corporation Housing waiting list, but like their sister and brother-in-law were told that it would be years before they had any chance of being housed. Cathie said, "I'm going back to the doctor to see if he will give me another letter regarding Jim's handicap". She continued..."I think he and Thomas need a room to themselves". "This big five apartment will be too big for the three of us, my Da, Ellen and me", said May, "we'll have to get a smaller house too", and she went back to reading her book. May still had her head always in a book. Granda said, "If the house fell round about us May will still carry on reading, and if we flit, the removal men will have to carry May out on her chair still reading her book". The conversation had given them all a lot to think about.

Cathie and Jimmy got ready to go home to be in on time for their visitors Vera and Willy, who usually did not come until nine o'clock. An odd time for anyone to go out and visit anyone, let alone take their daughter out at that time of night, thought Cathie.

That night in bed Cathie tossed and turned. She lay awake for hour after hour, try as she could she could not get to sleep. Soon after the light had gone out she could hear Tibby the cat doing his job of chasing the nice, and she thought that she could hear him catch one and was playing with it. This made her blood creep as she thought about it. She began to say her prayers and half way through the rosary she could hear the nice being chased by the cat again, "its a busy night for you tonight Tibby". She made up her mind, "I'm definitely going up to the doctor to get another line for the Corporation Housing Department in the morning. Oh' my God, I've got my turn of thewash-house in the morning. I'll have to get up early to stoke up and start the boiler and get the washing done first, and get it hung out. I hope it stays dry, at this rate it will be the morning before I get to sleep", she finally dossed off and got a few hours sleep.

The next morning she got up, still feeling very tired from lack of sleep, but Cathie knew that she had a lot to do. She went over and looked out of the window. "Thank God it's dry, and it looks like the sun might come out". So as Jimmy and the boys were still asleep, Cathie went out to the wash-house and got the fire going under the big stone boiler with sticks and rolled up newspapers. Now I better get in and get them ready, and get the breakfast, "Right boys, rise and shine, come on now its time to get up. I want to go to the surgery to ask the doctor if he will give me a line for the housing department for Jim's infantile paralysis". After a long wait in the surgery, Cathie went into see the doctor when her turn came. He knew all about Jim's case, and Cathie told him all about their housing situation. She then took the medical certificate up to the housing department. After a long wait there to see one of the housing officers, he told her that it would be between ten and twenty years before they would be able to house them. Cathie felt very depressed and fed-up at hearing this as she went home. As Thomas was still very small for his age, Jim could still get him into the boot at the back of his tricycle, and take him for a ride around the block of houses. By this time Jackie had got a tricycle the same as Jim's, and one day Margaret and Big John came up to visit with Jackie, who had his tricycle with him and young Frankie. While the adults were in the house the boys had a race on their tricycles with Thomas and Frankie sitting in the back, Jackie went over a bump and his young brother fell out and cut his head.

Chapter Nine
Up In The World

The two couples, Cathie and Jimmy, and Margaret and Big John, desided to buy small flats, and were very excited at the prospect of being owner-occupiers. The next day they went to the newsagents and bought all the morning and evening newspapers that advertised flats and houses for sale. They were looking for flats in the west-end of the city, at a price that they could afford. They went through the property pages taking notes of the flats that they would like to go and view. This was the start of an arduous task, which was both time consuming and also an education, as they had never dealt in this part of the housing market before. Margaret and Big John, who were worried about the amount of finance involved, told Cathie and Jimmy that they would wait to see how they got on. Jimmy said to them, "don't you worry, I will loan you the money for the deposit and any other expenses incurred.

Cathie and Jimmy went to view flats in the Whiteinch and Partick districts of the city. They wanted to be near the main road, the tramcars and the buses, and also the shops. They went to factors' offices, and got keys to go and view various one room and kitchen flats. The first set of keys that they got was for a flat up in the "Gangway", which was a "nickname" for an old gray sand-stone building. "And that's not very nice for a start!" said Cathie, "I would like to live in a red sand-stone building, Jimmy, with a bathroom". The Gangway was a dirty old gray building. It had a turret staircase and they had outside toilets on the landings.

The stairs at the back of the building led to each landing and to a walk-way with railings which ran along the back of the building. The main doors of some of the houses where off this walk-way. "No, I don't fancy Whiteinch either" was Jimmy's reply after Cathie had asked his opinion. "Come on then, I've got keys for a couple of flats that we will have to go and view in Partick", said Cathie. "Hurry-up then and we'll catch a tramcar into Partick", said Jimmy. "We better not take too long, the boys will be thinking that we have got lost", replied Cathie. "Oh, don't worry, you are worrying too much about these boys" Jimmy told her. They got down to the tramcar stop. "Good here is a car coming, timed that nice", said Jimmy. as they got on and paid their fair. "We'll try Partick", said Jimmy. "Aye, Partick sounds great to me" replied Cathie. As the tramcar went on its way along Dumbarton Road, she continued, "Look at all the shops, a great shopping area, everything I want right on hand; and even if you aren't going to buy anything, it will be great to go out for a walk and window shop; and you can get a tramcar and even a subway into the city centre", "Aye, and don' forget all the picture halls in Partick, and she began, "You've got The Rosevale, The Tivolia, The Partick Picture Hall, and don't forget The Western and The Standard, up at Partick Cross. All those halls right on your doorstep. Just think five picture halls with a change of program every three nights". "You don't like the pictures that much", Jimmy said to her. "Aye, but I like a good sad story with Allan Ladd", she replied and continued..."I like a good American picture, especially if it's in colour, but I don't like those British second pictures in black and white". Then Cathie thought of all the pubs that were in Partick, one on practically every corner. ""That will be too much of a temptation for you, and you know what you are like with the drink". "Oh, I've changed", said Jimmy. Cathie had heard that before, and wanted to believe it, but somehow in her heart she couldn't. She knew that she had to put it to the back of her mind, for the sake of the boys.

They arrived at their destination and descended from the tramcar. They proceeded to walk along the road to find the first flat that they wanted to view, then another and another. They met their sister-in-law, Mary, who lived in Partick, and Cathie and she had a wee blether. Cathie loved a wee gav (chat). "Oh, that will be great if you come to live in Partick, we'll see more of you", she said. "I thought that you were in a hurry, and worried about the boys" cried Jimmy. So they went on their way to have a look at the flats, one was too expensive, "They are asking too much for this" said Cathie. "They'll never get it sold, not at this price, they will have to drop the asking price if they want to get it sold", Jimmy added. The next flat that they went to see was a dump. "It would cost a fortune to do this place up, and you can smell the dry-rot and dampness, and its got woodworm, we'll definitely give this one a miss". "Yes, the close and stairs give me the creeps", Cathie said. They went on to view the last flat on their list. It was a one room, kitchen and bathroom, and it was in a red-sand-stoned building, she wanted. It was in a prominent location, near Partick Cross and the underground station. There was only one thing that they disliked about the flat, it was up four flights of stairs on the top landing. They went into the close from the street, and walked up one flight of stairs, which took them to the. back-court. The back-court was situated on the roof of the back of the ground floor shop, and the drying area was concrete, and had poles for the washing lines and a big midden. The high wall surrounding the back-court would make it safe enough for the boys to play in, thought Cathie. They then proceeded to go up the stairs. As they got to the first landing they noticed the lovely varnished hand-rail on the bannister and black painted shiny railings. Each flat had a lovely door with a stained-glass window, and they also had storm doors that had a lovely varnished finish, and brass handles and letter boxes which had been polished to give them a lovely shine. On the landing was the most beautiful stained glass window. "Fancy having these on the landing", they said to each other. "You think you are in church, they are lovely with the sun shining through them", said Cathie.

At last they reached the top landing. "Its a bit of a climb", said Jimmy, as they got to the top landing. "I like the red pipeclay on the landing and stairs, it gives it a nice rich effect, doesn't it". They looked at the names on the other two doors on the landing as they put the key into the lock of the storm door and opened it, to find the inner door, with the beautiful stained glass window on it, and also the brass handle and letter box. "If we take this house we will have to get a nice new brass name plate to go with them", said Jimmy. As they opened the door and went into the L shaped lobby, they saw the coal bunker sitting straight in front of them. "God help the coalman who has to carry bags of coal up all these stairs", said Cathie. She always made sure that the bunker was always well stocked up in case the coalman did not come, she would order two bags a week from the Co-op. "Nice wee lobby, I like the cornice. What size are the other flats on the landing ?" asked Jimmy. "A two room and kitchen and bathroom on the other side, and there is a small one room and kitchen and bathroom in the middle and then there is us" replied Cathie. "Us, does that mean that we're taking the house?" asked Jimmy "Aye well, wait till we see the rest, and we get the report from the surveyor"., said Cathie. The house had been unoccupied for sometime. The last occupant had died in the house and had been found behind the door, and there was a very fusty smell. There was also a lot of dirt and dust everywhere. Then the walked through to the front room. This was used as a living room and bedroom combined, and was a very big room with oriel windows, and as the sun was shining, Cathie remarked that it was a glow of light. The three windows, one facing south to the River Clyde, and beyond, another to the east with a good view of Partick Cross. The other window offered a good view down Dumbarton Road to the west. "It's a glow of light", Cathie kept saying as she surveyed the rest of the room. There is a big cupboard by the side of the window, where Jim can keep his toys and books, and Thomas will be able to keep his toys on the bottom shelves and on the floor as it will be easy for him to get them. The woodwork had a lovely grain and was beautifully varnished, like the lobby. They especially liked the mantlepiece, which had lovely carvings around the edging's. It also had nice tiles with figures like angles on them. It also had a tiled hearth and kerb. This room also had a lovely cornice around the walls and light, but it needed decorating. The room also had a big bed recess, and Cathie remarked that there was not a broken tile on the fire-place, which really pleased her. "Come on, come and see what the kitchen is like". They went through the lobby and opened the door to the kitchen. As they went in they could see that the kitchen, with its window looking out to buildings at the back of the flat was a different story, but, it did have potential. The big black range, with its oven, fire and stove would have to come out, along with the dirty old black sink with its old brass taps, but it did have running hot and cold water. The back boiler would also have to be lowered, and maybe even replaced; "It would be great to get hot boiling water for washing the clothes and for baths from the taps instead of having to boil water on the gas stove in the kettle and pots" said Cathie. "Aye, talking about baths, come-on-in and see the bathroom. Look at the size of the bath, its bigger than ma Da's It will take a lot of water to fill that up. Aye, it's big enough for two. We could have a bath together when the wains are in bed sleeping, or when Jim is staying down at his Granda's" said Jimmy. "Cut that out, we'll have none of that, you can forget that idea" said Cathie. The bathroom also had a big toilet pan with a high cistern and a dirty big black wooden seat on the pan. "that will really need a right good clean, no, better get a new one" said Cathie, who was spotlessly clean, about her home and family. The walls in the bathroom had wood panelling half way up and it to was varnished and had a lovely finish. The bathroom also had a lovely stained glass window at the top and frosted glass at the at the bottom. By this time both Cathie and Jimmy had fallen in love with the house, and were excited about buying it and moving in. But they knew that they had a lot of hard work in front of them, and a lot of expence. They took the keys of the flat back to the factor, and told him that they were interested in putting a bid for the flat, once the surveyor had past it. The factor told them that £300 was the asking price for the flat, but it would go to the highest offer, if there was more than one interested party. A couple of days passed, and Cathie and Jimmy were eager to get the surveyors report. It arrived in due course and he had past the flat for sale, and as no one else was interested in buying the flat they got it at the asking price of £300.

The followen day Cathie and Jimmy got up early, and after a hurried breakfast, they saw Jim off to school. They took Thomas down to Margaret, who was going to look after him while they went back to the factor and solicitors office in the city centre, as Jimmy had to sign the title-deeds and settle the financial agreement.

After they left the office with the keys, they felt very happy, and they could hardly wait to go and have another look at the flat that they had just bought. "We better go and get a bite to eat first, and I'm dying for a cup of tea", said Cathie, to which Jimmy replied, "I could go a pint". "Later", Cathie replied. They went to the City Bakers and had a cup of tea and something to eat. Then they got the tramcar to Partick and went up to see their house.

As they went up the close, with the keys of their own home, Jimmy said "This is great, wonderful", to which Cathie replied, "I can't believe that we are oner-occupiers", "Yes, we're really going up in the World". They went up the close to have another look at the back-court, and then up to the first landing, each time they stopped to read the name on the nameplate of each door that they passed on the way up the stair. At last they reached the top flat – it was four stories up. "I'm jiggered, it didn't seem as tiring the last time we came up". "It's four up, you know, but we'll get sued to it" said Cathie. "Well have to, we've bought the house". "Aye, your right there", was the reply.

They opened the doors and went into their flat. They had a much closer look round than they had the last time. "We are going to be busy, there is a lot of hard work ahead of us, and its going to take time", said Jimmy, and he continued "We won't move in until we have everything done". They were both hard workers and would not waste any time on getting on with the job. As Jimmy worked in the building trade before he had the accident, he had known where to buy material that they would need, plaster, bricks, etc. He asked his brother-in-law, who had a plumbers shop, and was also a plumber to trade if he could help him. There was not a pick on wee Bill, but he too was a grafter (hard worker). Once they got the tools of their trades up to the flat and the material that they needed the got stuck-in. They proceeded to pull out the old range, and as they did half the plaster and bricks on the wall came down, covering all with dust and soot; "For "F" sake, what a bloody mess". As they began to clean it up they said to each other, "this job is going to take a lot longer than we thought". "I got a good discount on the material from the suppliers" said Jimmy. After they had got the big black range out they had to lower the back boiler, and put in new pipes to enable them to get hot water from the fire in the new interior grate that they were going to put in. Cathie and Jimmy had bought a lovely new interior grate fireplace, and the tiles were really nice. "One thing at a time, we'll get this done first, the fire in, and check the hot water supply, and then we'll go to work on the sink", said Bill.

Once that they saw that the hot water supply was running alright, and to Bill's satisfaction, they set to work on the sink. It was an old black sink and it had old fashioned brass taps that looked very dirty. They were very hard to turn on and off, and the draining board was also pot black as well as worn, with the wood being washed and scrubbed over the years. A new white wally sink accompanied with new chrome taps had been delivered, and Bill installed them. The new taps were marked H & C for hot and cold running water. While they had been at the supplies, Cathie noticed tin or stainless steel material that could be cut to size to cover the draining-board, and she thought that it would have a nice finish, and enhance the finish of her kitchen. Jimmy and Bill then took off the door of the cupboard by the side of the fire and also took out the shelves and plastered up the wall. They put the stainless steel up around the wall before they installed the new gas cooker that Cathie and Jimmy had bought form the Gas Board. "Well, that's all the main jobs done, thank God," "Aye, I thought we would never get it done", said the pair of them together !

Next for the decorating. "We'll need to go to the wallpaper shop and buy the wallpaper and paint that we need to get the house done up". "As the doors and windows are varnished, we won't have to buy any gloss paint, but we need emulsion for the ceilings and wallpaper for the walls. I'd like a real nice paper for the room, something white with a nice gold flower or leaf. I saw something in the shop that I like, and nice curtains to match. Aye, I've got an idea, wall-lights, it would be a good idea to get wall-lights up on the wall above the fire-place, and one in each of the bed recesses, to let us had a read in bed and you won't have to get up to put the light off" said Cathie. "I know an electrician who is always looking for "homers" and he will be glad to do the job, and it shouldn't take that long". "What will you think of next ?" "That's it, I think we have covered everything". "Oh' no we haven't said Cathie. "What do you mean ?" asked Jimmy. "The walls, we have'ny covered the walls", and with a laugh Cathie continued, "We had better go and buy that wallpaper and paste and the other things that we need".

"It's good that we don't have to worry about the boys. I know that they are getting well looked after while we get on with the work", Cathie said, as they went off to buy the wallpaper and paint. It took them a couple weeks, but it was worth al the hard work, it looked really lovely when it was finished, so clean and bright, it was worth all the hard work. They even varnished the woodwork surrounds to give it a nice fresh finish as it needed freshening up, and also the floor surrounds in the room as they had bought a lovely big carpet for the centre of the floor. There was a sale on at the Co-op, and they got a really good bargain. They also went out and bought a three-piece suite, made of rexceen, an imitation leather, with a fold up bed in the couch, and as they liked the thought of owning a piano, they went out and bought one. Although neither of them could play, they thought that it would be good exercise for Jim's shaking hands.

At last the house was ready and the day of the flitting had arrived. Everything went smothely, and they all settled in to spend the first night in their new home. That night they lit a fire in the grate in the kitchen, and there was plenty of hot water and they could all have a lovely bath.

Margaret and Big John had also been looking for a small flat in thePartick district of the city. They found a one room and kitchen with an inside toilet on the ground floor of a tenement building, just about half a mile from where Cathie and Jimmy lived. It was at a price that they could afford. They went through the procedure of buying the flat, and put down a deposit and would pay the remainder by monthly installments. They too got the flat decorated and moved in. It was a smaller room and kitchen than their sister and brother-in-law's, and only had an inside toilet. However, Margaret and Big John were delighted with their first home of their own after seven years of married life. It was low down in the close, which Margaret liked as she could keep on eye on the boys as they were out playing in the back-court, and she could have a wee blether to her neighbours through the kitchen window as she did her washing and peeled her potatoes and vegetables in the sink. By God, Margaret could talk, and sometimes she forgot to go and get her messages in, and would ask Jackie, or Jim is he was along after school to go to the ships and get the messages in on time for John's tea when he came home from work. There was a good chippy down the street and Jackie would go and get a fish supper for his Daddy and bags of chips, or a pie or black pudding supper for his Mammy and the children. Sometime Big John got fed up with chips, and would say, "No bloody chips again, I'll turn into a bloody chip or a fish". They were a happy couple, and Margaret idolized Big John and he thought the world of her.

Granda's big five apartment had become too much for him and his two remaining daughters, who were unmarried and still lived in the house with him. The rent was too much for them, and the house had become too much for Ellen to keep clean. It was also becoming far to big an unkeep, especially with so many rooms to heat, they had bit bills for coal and gas.

Granda, May and Ellen agreed that they should look for a smaller house, and Ellen went to the corporation housing department to ask if they could have a mutual exchange, or an offer of a smaller house. The corporation offered her a move to a one room and kitchen, kitchenette and bathroom. She took the keys and went to view the house, and then talked Granda and May into taking the house and got Granda to go and sign the missive. Cathie and Margaret told Ellen that she should have waited until she could have got a three apartment, and added that in their opinion, she acted in haste, but Ellen thought of the cheap rent, and the money that she would save from the house-keeping, and moved before the 28th of that month to save her paying an extra months rent.

They got help from the rest of the family to flit, and to help with the laying of the floor covering. They had to get rid of some of the furniture as it would not all fit into the smaller house. Cathie went down to help her sisters get things sorted out. Molly, an older cousin, came down to paper the living-come-bedroom. She was very good with her hands and she was also very good with a paste brush and paint brush. Molly went into the kitchenette to mix the wallpaper paste. At the same time, Ellen was peeling the potatoes for Granda's and May's dinner, she was making mince and tatties. Molly noticed that Ellen was cutting the skin's off the potatoes too thick, and said, "Ellen, you are cutting half the tatties away". Ellen was so angry that she threw a potato at Molly, who said "your mince is far too watery, its like hot water with mince floating on top of it", thee was a heated exchange. Not such an amicable start to the new surroundings.

Their house was looking nice. It suited Ellen with May out at work all day and Granda out all day too It gave Ellen the run of the house to herself during the day, and she would go and sell anything that she could to the ragman, or take anything that she could to the ragstore to get extra money to go to the dancing, and the ragman came along the street almost every other day with his horse and cart. If she got enough money she would go to the dancing up in the Playhouse Ballroom in the afternoon and again in the evening, sometimes five times a week. She liked to dance to the music of Doctor Crock and his Crackpots, and would take great pleasure in telling Jim and Jackie all about it when they went down to visit.

Cathie and Margaret and their families had settled nicely into their new homes. They took great pride in keeping their homes spick and span. They always cleaned in every corner. Cathie would always say that it was not just the places that could be seen that had to be kept clean, but the corners and under the beds in the bed recesses also had to be kept clean. The bed recesses were great for keeping things like cases and baths and toolboxes under. They also found them a great place to hide the children's toy, as they bought them before Christmas. Cathie always kept the toys well hidden from Jim and Thomas, and they did not see them until Christmas Eve, and then they would bring them out and put them under the big Christmas tree thay she dought from the Co-operative fruiters, and she and Jimmy also bought a set of Christmas tree lights. They must have been one of the few homes in Glasgow to have lights on their Christmas tree in 1952. Jim and Thomas and Jackie and Frankie were delighted when they saw them. "Ah, their wee faces are all lit up", said Margaret. Margaret would show the boys were the toys were hidden, and open the boxes of sweets and take some out, and tell the boys not to say anything. She was very sweet mouthed, and took some of the sweets out to eat, and said that she could put them back later, before Santa Claus came on Christmas Eve.

Cathie and Margaret visited each others home almost every day. They saw Jimmy and Big John off to work, and Jim and Jackie off to school. After they had made their pieces and gave them their breakfast. Usually Jimmy got himself out. But Cathie always got up for Jim, to help him get ready and go down and see him safely across the busy road to get the school bus. Jim stood to wait for the bus with another two boys.

Bit John had changed his job. He had left his job as a coalman, and he had got a job as a labourer in shipyard on Clydeside in the west-end of the city. Sometimes he would get sent away on the ships for sea-tials, and be way for weeks. Margaret did not mind this as he got a lot of extra money, and it always came in handy for getting things for their home.

He was still a good footballer, playing in the Scottish Junior league, and was getting some money fron that, which also helped them to get things for the house. His team got to the finals of the Scottish Junior Cup, and Big John was very pleased to play at Hampden Park, as he had told Margaret that it had always been one of his ambitions, along with playing for one of the big clubs in Scotland. He also told her that he had always hoped that a scout would spot him and give him a trail, but thought that he was getting too old for that now. "Never mind", Margaret told him. "You have made it to the final, and we are all going to the game to support you". On the day of the cup final Big John left early to go and join his team. Ellen came up and looked after Thomas and Frankie as they were too young to go to the big game. The rest of the family all went along to cheer Big John and his team on. Big Johns' mother had a tear in her eye as she watched her son playing. Jim and Jackie were very excited to be in the main stand, as were Margaret and Cathie, who had their photograph taken, and Margaret was interviewed by a newspaper reporter. Who asked her how she felt about her husband playing. When the game started they cheered Big John and his team on until they were hoarse. They had all planned to go to a big celebration if his team won, but they lost 1-0. Everyone was very sad and disappointed as they went on their way home. "Never mind John", said Margaret, "You did get to play in the final, and you have always got your medal".

Jimmy's legs had got a lot better, and the doctor had signed him off the sick panel as being fit for light work. He could walk unaided by his walking stick. He went along to the broo (employment exchange) to see what they had to offer him as he could not go back to his old trade as it would be far too dangerous for him. At that time they had plenty of jobs on offer, and some people were changing their jobs all the time. After a series of interviews he got a position as a storeman in a large engineering firm. They had a lot of orders, and he worked day shift and night shift on a month about rota. He also got a lot of overtime. Cathie was delighted that he had started work again, and was glad to get him out of the house from under her feet all day, and if he went out, she had the worry of him coming home drunk, for he always met someone in the pub. He said to her when he brought home his first pay, "Cathie, its good to be working again". "Yes", she replied, "as long as you come home for your tea, and stay off the drink". He handed her the housekeeping money, which he had taken out of the pay packet, along with his own spending money and threw the pay packet away before he got home. He did not want Cathie to know how much he earned, and that he had as much to spend on himself as she had from him to keep the house. She had to "scrimp and scrape" at the end of the week to make ends meet. She was a good manager and always got by on what he gave her, just. But, he always seemed to have plenty of money in his pocket, and could always go to the match, even the mid-week match and go for a drink afterwards. Cathie told him that she did not mind him going to the football, or even going for a pint after the game as long as he didn't come back home drunk. That was the thing that she dreaded most, and so did Jim.

Chapter Ten
HISTORICAL TIMES

While he was down visiting his Granda and auntie's house, Jim's cousin , Jackie also came to visit. They had Sunday lunch with Granda, Auntie May and Ellen. Auntie May always cooked the meals at the weekend, and she was a good cook, so Jim and Jackie always eat their meal. They hated their Auntie Ellen's cooking, her gravey was like boiled water, and half the time she forgot to salt the food. They also did not like her sandwiches, as she put a dollop of butter in the middle of a slice of bread and forgot to spread it. She would forget to stir the custard and it would be put onto the table lumpy. Jim said to his Auntie May, "I'm glad you made dinner, we can eat it when you cook, we can'y eat Auntie Ellen's cooking, her custard and rice are like wallpaper paste, all lumpy and goey". Auntie Ellen was not at all pleased with this remark, and "blew her top" and a big argument developed between the two of them. Auntie Ellen called Jim "twitchy face". That has always stuck in Jim's mind.

They went off to the cemetery to visit her Granny's grave and put flowers on it, which they bought from a lady selling them at the entrance. The main purpose of the visit as far as the boys were concerned, well was too-fold, to visit the grave of their Granny, and the cafe up the road to get an ice or a drink!

When they arrived they put the flowers on the grave and knelt down to say a prayer for their Granny's soul – that it would go to heaven, and that she would be with God. Auntie May tidied up the grave and took the boys on a tour of all the other relatives that had died in the past, most of whom the boys had never heard of. By this time they were decidedly fed-up, and only wanted to get to the cafe, and then home.

On the way home the tramcar stopped and the two cousins and their auntie had to get off at their stop. The tramcar lines were in the middle of the road and an Orange Walk, to celebrate King Billy and the Battle of the Boyne, with flute bands and pipe bands playing, and banners flying, the two boys not thinking, ran through it. A woman in the march shouted at them.

Auntie May and the two cousins finally got across the road to catch another tramcar home. Jim was the first to get off the tramcar at his stop. He ran along the road to his close, and up the stair to the door of the house and banged on it. Cathie opened the door, and everyone was in the kitchen, and the front room was in darkness. Jim went in, switched on the light, although it was still daylight and went over to the dressing-room table which had a mirror. It sat in the oriel window. He looked into the mirror and he spoke to himself to see if his mouth was twitchy. He did it again, and again, just to make sure, and it was. He took out his comb and combed his hair, and thought to himself, "Ah well, I suppose I'm not too bad looking", and with a wee laugh, he put it to the back of his mind.

At school Jim began to be given cookery lessons. At first he thought, cookery was for girls and cissys. As the lessons progressed, however he began to enjoy making soup, baked apple and cakes, and taking home samples for his family to taste. They always found them delicious. Also at school, Jim and his class were reading Scottish history. He loved to read of the Picts and the Celts, and of the battles between the clans of Scotland. Miss Doughtery made the lesson come to life. This gave Jim a pride in Scotland, and he thought that it should be a separate nation. In geography the children learned that Scotland was part of Great Britian and all the pink land on the map of the World belonged to them. This got Jim thinking, "to belong is to be part of, or to own". How can we own another country ?

Their next door neighbour, Old Kate, began to wander, due to old age, and Cathie began to get very worried about her. She told her family of her concern. They asked Cathie to keep an eye on her, which she did.

She was very attentive, and took her out every day to get her messages, and for walks to Kelvingrove Park.

Old Kate began to go out for walks during the night. She would come to Cathie's door during the night wanting to go out to the shops. Eventually she had to go into hospital to be looked after properly. While Old Kate was in hospital, Cathie still went in to check on old Joe, Katie's husband, who had a bad leg and could not go out. She got his messages and asked the coalman to bring up his bags of coal. His family still came up to visit him, but it was not easy for them as they did not stay near-by. After a few months in hospital old Kate died, and everyone was very sad. Her body was brought home and put in her room. Everyone went in that night to say the rosary. Old Kate lay in her coffin in her bedroom, which was through the wall from Jim's bedroom. That made him feel very, very eerie! As Old Kate had a very small house, Cathie offered to let her family have the funeral in her big front room, and they were delighted to accept. Cathie and Jimmy got a nice spread laid out on the table of sandwiches, sausage rolls and cakes, and there was plenty of refreshments —beer, whisky, tea and coffee. Cathie got up early and attended the requiem mass, and then come home to have things ready for the return of the mourners from the cemetery.

Old Kate had quite a large family and a lot of friends. It was a very wet and windy day, and Cathie told Jim that a wet day for a funeral meant that the dead person was happy, and had a happy death. Jim thought, "happy death, I don't see anyone laughing!" The mourners began to return from the cemetery, and were soaked to the skin. Everyone was very hungry and dry after they had been out all morning and the food and drink was quickly consumed. Some people began to get a little bit tipsy, and the guests began to leave after a couple of hours. After they had all gone, Cathie said, "Thank God that's over", then she said to Jimmy, "Oh' no, look at that, someone has burned a hole in the arm of our good rexeen settee, with a cigarette,, and just look at the mess of my carpet. There is a cigarette burn in it too. It is just as well that our house is insured for contents as well as building", she said, and continued, "everyone should have their home insured, you never know when you might need it".

It was 1953 and television had begun to broadcast in central Scotland a year earlier. It was proving to be quite popular with the public, and people and the press were predicting that many cinemas would close down as a result of people buying sets. However the high price of £60 to £90 put a lot of people off buying a set as it was way beyond their means. Cathie and Margaret liked to take the boys out for a walk along Dumbarton Road to look in at the television sets that were on in the shop windows, to see the sometimes flickering pictures that appeared on the screens. The Stand Cafe had a set, and Jim liked to go over with his wee brother and his Mammy to see the "wireless with pictures" T.V. It was always an excuse to get his Mammy to buy him an ice drink.

The Queen was to be crowned in June at her coronation at Westminster Abbey in London. Flags and bunting were being put up in every city, town and village in Britian and all over the commonwealth – and Glasgow – and everywhere was looking nice, bright and clean for a change. Cathie, and about every other housewife, was giving her windows an extra wash, and buying new curtain material to make new curtains. She put pictures of The Queen and The Duke of Edinburgh in the window. Street parties were arranged in almost every street, and the picture hall also had parties for the children of their regular patrons. Jim went to a party in the Western Picture Hall and enjoyed it very much, as the children got ice cream, sweets and bottles of soft drinks, and a tin of sweets to take home. He also went round the corner to enjoy a street party, where the children sat at long tables which were put out out along the middle of the street and laiden with goodies for the children with sandwiches and cakes, fruit and sweets and lemonade. All the children got party hats and flags to wave as they sang and danced to records that someone played from a record-player sitting on their window ledge, with the volume turned up full. Street entertainers were also in attendance to sing and dance and tell jokes that most of the children had already heard! A street party was held in the evening, when the adults a drink and a dance. As Jim was getting washed and ready for his bed he heard reports of the days events on the wireless, and also that Hillory had with Shepard Tenson conquered Everest. Jim asked, "Who's Everest?" and was told, "Mount Everest is the Worlds highest mountain".

One day not long after the Queen's Coronation Jim came home from school to a wonderful surprise. Cathie opened the door to him and told him to close his eyes and go into the front room. "Hold your hands over your face, and don't look until I tell you", she told him. Jim covered his eyes with his hands and he knew that he was in for some kind of surprise, but could not think what it might be.

Along the small lobby he proceeded to walk until he reached the door of the front room, which Cathie opened. They went in. In front of him, by the side of the fireplace stood a mahogany cabinet with two doors with handles. Jim was speechless, then said "a television, we have a television, this is one of the happiest days of my life". Cathie could laughed. Jim went over and opened the doors to reveal a 12 inch screen, a speaker, and four knobs. Yes, it was a television, the thing that Jim had been longing for since he saw them at the exhibition. "There is nothing on", said Cathie, "Have you any homework to do?" she asked him. "If you have you better get it done before children's house starts at five o'clock" she continued. "The television comes on for an hour, and then it goes off again until eight, when programs for grown-ups come on. "Can I see some of them later ?" Jim asked. "If you are good and eat your dinner" replied his Mammy. Just then the door bell rang, and it was Auntie Margaret with her two boys, she too came into the room. "Oh my God, Cathie, when did you get that? It must have cost a bomb, have you won the pools or something ?" she asked. "It's a 12 inch Phillips consul model, we got it from the shop across the road. You need an aerial. We have a socket in this room, and one in the kitchen as well, and I can wheel it through if I want to watch it in there", said Cathie. "You must be loaded paying that kind of money. I could think of better things to do with it, like rig-oot the wanes", said Margaret. "You could get the wanes rigged-oot from head to toe, and buy a good rig-oot for yourself with that money, and still have something left over to buy something for the house. I like nice ornaments for the hoose, Aye, I like nice ornaments". She went on "Do you know, I saw a lovely pair of wally dugs in a shop just along the road, but they're just too dear, Ah' just couldn'y afford them. Anyway never mind that, turn the thing on and let's see what happens". Jim turned on the switch, and the test card came on. "Well, at least it goes, and I'm ding for a cup of tea" said Margaret as she and Cathie went into the kitchen.

5 o'clock, and the children's programmes began. Cousin John was in the house. "Want to see the television?" Jim asked John as they went into the room to view a puppet show. Jim thought that it was very enjoyable, but John said "That's kids stuff".

Everyone was making an excuse to come to visit, and see the television. Cathie's tea pot was never off the gas, and it was costing her a fortune in tea, milk and sugar, not to mention bread and butter and biscuits and cakes. If it was someone that they had not seen for a while, Cathie would send out for fish suppers. But, she did not complain, as she and Jimmy both liked company. But, she said to him, "this is costing me a packet, the money is hardly lasting out the week; I could be doing with a bit more in my housekeeping money".

Every night it was always the same, people arriving before transmission began, and some would stay until the wee white dot had vanished from the screen. They watched anything and everything, as there was only one channel. Adults like "Andy Pandy", with Looby Loo and Little Ted, and "Muffin the Mule" and the Newsreel – long plays that they did not understand and the Proms! Margaret loved the Proms, especially when Malcolm Sargent was conducting, and the quiz shows, "What's my line?" and "Animal, Vegetable or Mineral". Then there was the cricket, boring old cricket. "I don't know how anyone could sit and watch that all day, it would put me to sleep", said Cathie.

Jim asked his Mammy one day if she was going to become a school teacher. Cathie said "That is a silly question, why are you asking me that ?" Jim replied that most of the teachers in his school were fat and wore a smock, and his Mammy was getting fat and was wearing a smock, but Cathie told him that it was just to keep her clothes clean as she did her housework.

A few months later Jim noticed that his Mammy was packing a small suitcase, and got it into his head that his Mammy had had enough of his Daddy drinking, and was planning to go away and leave him and his wee brother with his Daddy. The thought of that terrified the life out of Jim. He worried about it to himself and wondered if his Mammy would still be at home when he returned home from school. Each day he gave a sigh of relief as he found that his mother was still at home.

One night Cathie told Jim and Thomas that she would have to go into hospital for a few days, but they were not to worry as she would be home soon and would bring them back something nice. Jim quizzed her as to what it might be, but all she would say was "Wait and see". Then she told them that their Auntie Ellen was coming to look after them; "Bloody Hell", said Jim. He had not forgotten the twitchy face incident.

That night Cathie, escorted by Jimmy, went off in a taxi to the hospital. Jim did not sleep much that night. He believed his Mammy, but still had worrying doughts in his mind that something was wrong.

The next morning, he awoke, after a few hours sleep, to the sound of his Daddy's voice in a loud roar, "Wakey, wakey" he shouted, "you have a new baby sister. "She is very nice, a lovely wee girl with blonde curly hair, I think, (he wasn't quite sure) six pounds something, and she is to be called Kathleen Anne. The two boys Jim and Thomas just looked at each other and said "Good", and turned over on their pillows and went to sleep. Jim felt a sense of relief that his Mammy would indeed becoming back home again. Later that day they were taken to the hospital to visit their Mammy and see their new baby sister. "She is very nice. Does she cry a lot ?" asked Thomas. "And, does she sleep at night ?" asked Jim. "I hope she sleeps a lot better that you did", his Mammy replied.

A few days later Cathie arrived home to a lovely welcome with the new baby, but she did not get much rest because she had to get on with her housework, and all the extra washing. The hospital staff had told Cathie to rest and take things easy when she got home. "That's easier said than Done" thought Cathie. "What's that my Ma used to say", "A woman's work is never done", she was right. I've only been home for a few days, and the washing is pilling up already. Then there is all the extra washing for the baby. That's one thing you can't let fall behind". After a rest and a cup of tea, she asked Ellen to take the boys to the park, and she proceeded to get some of her washing done at the sink for she knew that she would need the sink again before tea-time to get the dinner on. Cathie did manage to get a couple of hours rest in the afternoon, and then it was back to normal. Get up feed and change the baby, peel the tatties, and get the rest of what was for dinner ready, and the table set. Then the two boys and their Auntie Ellen came back from the park. "We're hungry, what's for dinner ?" shouted the boys as they arrived from playing on the swings and having a walk. Then Jimmy arrived home from his work and they all sat down to have their meal. They were very happy all that week. The baby was a good wee sleeper, although Cathie still had to get up for the two o'clock feed.

Then the following Friday morning, as he was about to leave for work, Jimmy said to Cathie, "I'll be a wee bit late tonight. I'm taking some of the lads out for a drink to wet the baby's head." Cathie replied

"What about my house-keeping money. Can you not bring that home first ? I need my wages to get extra messages in-case we get visitors to see the baby, I've had a lot of extra expense this week. Why don't you come home first and have your dinner, and wash and change, and then go out with the lads ? You'll feel a lot better, and so will I." He did not answer and left for work and Cathie began her daily routine.

Jimmy did come home from work and they all had a lovely dinner. "Are you still going out? We are having visitors to see the baby" Cathie told him. "I won't be long, just a couple of hours" Jimmy replied as he left for the pub. He did arrive home, very, very late, and very much the worst for drink. He was in a very bad temper. He staggered against the door, and into the kitchen, knocking everything over, that was in his way, he demanded his meal, and when it was on the table, he did not eat it. "You missed the visitors, and that's a terrible way to come home" said Cathie. He staggered from the table, throwing his arms about, and then knocked Jim against the door. Jim lost his temper and gave his Daddy a kick on the leg. Then Jimmy made a dive for Jim and fell onto the pram nearly knocking the baby out. At this Cathie got really angry and tried to get her wages out of his pocket, as he shouted that he was going out for more drink. Cathie told him that he had enough drink for one night, and that he would be better in his bed. Jimmy made a dive for Cathie, and began to punch her. Wee Jim tried to intervene to save his mother. Wee Jim got punched very hard and fell over, and hurt himself. This made Cathie even more angry, as Jimmy continued his cursing and swearing, as he made to hit Cathie again. He made his way over to the sink, and took of his shirt and began to wash the top half of his body and hair, still shouting very loudly, and throwing punches as Cathie told him to be quiet. With his head and top half of his body covered in soap suds, he punched Cathie again, and by this time she was hysterical. Cathie lost control and lifted a pint of milk that had been standing on the draining board and hit Jimmy over the head with it. It was just like an explosion in an ice-cream factory, with the milk, shampoo and blood it looked just like ice-cream and raspberry. All hell was let lose and Jimmy went berserk again. The police were called and Jimmy was taken away. As he was taken away he was still shouting and swearing.

The following morning the new baby was to be christened up in the chapel after the twelve o'clock Mass, and Ellen was to be her Godmother.

This made Ellen very proud, as she was not Godmother of two children. She would say that she was a Fairy-Godmother, and Jim said "I don't know about that, but she is certainly away with the fairies". Cathie got up very early to get the boys, the new baby and herself ready, and the christening piece was made up. She was still feeling ill after all that had happened the previous night and was worrying about what Jimmy might do. She was in two minds. She did not know whether to bail him out or leave him until Monday.

Ellen arrived and they all left for the chapel. As they walked up the road they met a young boy and gave him the christening piece. They arrived at the chapel. Cathie said "Sit at the back until the end of Mass in case the kids misbehave". Ellen said" I hope it is not the old parish priest, he goes on, and on. At the end of Mass, after all the congregation had left the chapel, a nice young priest that Cathie and Ellen liked came down and baptised the baby Kathleen Anne in the baptismal font at the back of the chapel, as Cathie, and her two sons looked on. Ellen said to Cathie, "You look terrible, like death warmed up". "So would you, if you had to experience what I had last night. Your lucky, your single". said Cathie, and she continued, "I wish I had stayed single, but still, I wouldn't part with my kids".

They sat down to Sunday dinner, but Cathie and Jim did not enjoy it, as they were worried about the thought of having to go to court and stand in the witness box.

At the court on the Monday morning they were very nervous, and young Jim was shaking like a leaf, even though Cathie had given him one of his pills. As wee Jim was too small to be seen or heard from the witness box the magistrate asked Jim to come up and stand on a chair beside him, to enable him to hear what Jim was saying. Jimmy was find and bound over to keep the peace. They all went home together, and made-up their differences. Jimmy went into his work late, but Jim got the rest of the day off from school to recover from his frightening ordeal.

Jimmy returned home from work in the evening and the family had a nice meal of Jim's favourite, mince and tatties, and they watched the television and had an early night. The were all happy again for months to come, but Cathie and wee Jim wondered, how long would it last.

It was Margaret's turn to go into hospital to have her third child, and she had a series of false alarms. Big John and she would go up to the hospital with Margaret's wee case, that had all been packed. On their way there, they stopped and Big John ran up to Cathie's house with their two boys, as Cathie had agreed that she would look after them while their Mammy was in the hospital. The boys thought that it was great staying together, and all sleeping in the same bed. It was an awful lot of work for Cathie, with the five children to look after, with them all being so young. But Cathie was well used to looking after a lot of children, and Jackie and Frankie were well used to her. It was not the children that Cathie worried about, but whether Jimmy would behave himself while their nephews were staying with them. Big John came up every evening for his dinner, to see his sons before he went to visit Margaret. He also came up on his way home from visiting Margaret in the hospital to let Cathie and Jackie and Frankie know how Margaret was getting on. "No news yet" he would say to Cathie as she opened the door to him every night. "My God, that baby is taking its time, she's a week over due already" said Cathie. After a quick cup of tea, Big John would make his way home, and as he left he said, "I wish she would hurry-up, I hate an empty house, I miss her and the boys". Margaret was detained in hospital for a few weeks because her blood pressure was high. She and big John had booked a single-end for a holiday in Anstruther in Fife, and she was worried that she would not have the baby in time as she was looking forward to her holiday, and did not want to cancel it at the last minute. As she lay in her bed in the maternity ward at night she prayed that her baby would come soon, and she could still go on holiday.

One morning Jimmy got up, took his bicycle, and set off for his work as usual. Cathie then got up and fed and changed the baby before getting Jim and Jackie up and after giving them breakfast saw them off to school. Once she had got baby Kathleen bathed and all changed and given her bottle, she put her down into her pram. Then after a sit down to a cup of tea and a wee fag, she had to get the porridge on again for Thomas and Frankie, the two younger boys, who were still fast asleep in bed. "Come on boys, rise and shine, time to get up, your porridge and orange juice is on the table. I have a lot to do today, and we must hurry-up and get ready to go to the ships, as I've got old Joe's messages to get as well as my own. We will have to go in and check on old Joe. He had not been keeping well since old Kate died, and isn't able to go out on his own now". After getting the children ready to go to the shops, Cathie went in to see what old Joe needed. "You should really eat more, Joe, I don't think your feeding yourself right since Kate died, don't let yourself go", she would scold him.

As Cathie went back into her own house to get her purse, it began to rain, and it got heavier by the minute. She told the boys to play with their toys until the rain went off, and she began to clean the house, beginning with the front room. She kept going into the kitchen to see that the baby was still asleep and check-up on the two boys to see what they were doing.

Baby Kathleen was sound asleep in her cot, and the two young boys were playing with their toy cars, and their Cowboy and Indians on the floor by the side of the bed recess, which had a valance curtain hanging from the side of the built-in-bed. The boys were quiet and contented as they played away with their toys an the only sound that Cathie heard coming from the kitchen was bang-bang, your dead, as Thomas and Frankie shot at and killed each-others cowboys and Indians. Unknown to Cathie the two boys had found a box of matches. One of the boys, neither would admit guilt, took out a match from the match box and struck a light. The light from the match set fire to the valance curtain, and soon the fire had spread to the curtains which hung down each side of the bed-recess, and onto the pelmet at the top. The two boys began to cry and scream hysterically, and as soon as Cathie heard this, she dropped everything and ran into the kitchen as fast as her legs could carry her. She was shocked by what she saw but she did not hesitate. She got hold of Thomas and Frankie by the arm and ran with them into old Joe's next door. Banging on his door, and shouting, "Fire, fire, fire" at the pitch of her voice. Old Joe opened the door as fast as he could, to find the two boys standing there on the landing, and smoke coming from Cathie's door. Then Cathie ran out of her house with the baby in her arms.

Cathie ran past old Joe shouting to get a neighbour to phone the fire brigade. A neighbour, Mr Smith, heard the loud shouts and came out of his house. He hurried back in and phoned the fire brigade. By this time Cathie had the baby safely tucked-up at the back of old Joe's bed, and she and old Joe were already tackling the fire by themselves, running in and out of the house with buckets of water which they got from old Joe's bathroom. Cathie and old Joe managed to get most of the fire out at the bed-recess by the time the fire brigade arrived. The fire officer told them that they had gone a good job. However, the fire had spread to the pully, which as usual was full of washing which Cathie had done the previous day. The firemen soon got the rest of the fire out. Then they congratulated Cathie and said that she had done a great job getting the boys out, and saving the baby.

They telephoned Jimmy at his work and asked him to come home, which he did. In the meantime Cathie went in to survey the damage that the fire had caused to her nice kitchen. She was feeling so sad that she shed a little tear. As she began to look around she saw the pully laying down, one end on the floor, the other end on top of the kitchen table, with the top part of Jimmy's good suit jacket pocket not burnt. Sticking out from the breast pocket was a pay-slip. Cathie could not believe her eyes, as she looked at it and saw that he had as much money to spend on himself, for cigarettes, football and drink as he was giving her to keep the house, pay all the bills and feed the children. She began to wonder if he really did have another woman somewhere, then she thought to herself, its definitely not that, no one else is daft enough to put up with him.

Although she was furious with him she decided not to say anything in the meantime, as they had enough on their hands with cleaning up after the fire, and getting the children fed, and the baby fed and changed. Her head was spinning. She didn't know where to start. Luckily the kitchen cabinet had not been burnt and there was food in it for dinner. The settee in the front room went down to a double bed, so the four boys could sleep in that, and we can sleep in the bed-recess, she decided.

Jim arrived home from school. As he was going up the close he could smell smoke, which seemed to get stronger the nearer he got to his house. He rang the bell and his Daddy opened the door. Jim got a shock when he saw that the walls in the lobby were all dirty and black, and the awful smell of smoke still lingered. "Bloody-Hell, what happened, has there been a fire ?" he asked. "You're very observant", replied his Daddy, as Jim asked "is the television O.K. ?" Jimmy shouted at Jim "Is that all you can think about, are you not concerned about your family, your wee brother and your wee sister and the rest of them". "Never mind that just now" said Cathie, and she continued "Jim, here is money and a list of messages and the message bag. You can go to the Co-op. You can go and get things that I need for tonight's tea, and get something for your Daddy's piece for his work tomorrow". "I had better take the morning off from work and go up to the insurance office and get a claims form. Aye, it is just as well we have our insurance" said Jimmy.

A newspaper reporter came up to the door looking for a story and wanted to interview them. He rang the door bell and wanted to ask Cathie some questions, just then another arrived on the landing. He was from another evening newspaper. "Is this the heroine who rescued the baby from the blazing cot ?" he asked. "I don't want any publicity, I'm up to my eyes in it, and my sister is in the hospital to have a baby. I don't want want her to see it in the papers in case she gets a fright. I want her husband to go up and tell her what happened himself, as she would be very worried, especially as I'm looking after her two sons", said Cathie. The reporters then went on their way. Sometime later Big John arrived for his dinner, and he too got the shock of his life. No one had telephoned his work to let him know what had happened. Cathie had had enough of her hands with the children and the cleaning up. He had gone straight to his own house to get washed and changed, before he came up for dinner.

"I don't trust these reporters. Away down and get all the evening papers, Jim, to see if there is anything in them", asked Cathie. Jim went down the stairs to the newsagents and bought all the evening papers. They all hurriedly read through the papers, and saw the headlines "City mother saves baby from blazing cot". "Hurry-up John, get to the hospital and tell Margaret what happened before she sees the newspaper and gets a fright".

Once Big John was off to visit Margaret, Cathie and Jimmy continued to clean-up as much as they could, and get the children washed and into their bed for the night. Cathie was absolutely livid every time that she thought about Jimmy's pay-slip.

On the mantelpiece, tucked behind the clock, and in front of a big pile of unopened mail was a buff envelope, which had arrived by post on the morning after the fire. Cathie had forgotten all about it, with the events of the day. All the activity had put it right out of her mind. She thought about Jimmy's wage slip. She was determined to challenge him about it, although she was dreading what his reaction would be like, although she had a good idea. She knew that he would "blow his top". But she was really fuming at the thought of him having a much money in his pocket to spend on his boozy pals in the pub, and going to see his beloved Partick Thistle, as she had to keep the house, pay all the bills, and feed and clothe the kids, "the bloody self-centered swine. Just wait till he comes in from his work he will have to do some very good explaining to get out of this one. He will not have an excuse, he will just have to cough up more money for the running of the house, or I'll not be here", Cathie would tell him, although she had know intention of leaving her kids. "What a fate for my poor weans, no way would I leave them with him, or anyone else."

The insurance assessor came up to that morning to assess the extent of the damage to the household effects, and had a good look round. Cathie gave him a list, and told him that a lot of things that had been destroyed had been of sentimental value. The insurance valuer said that he would go away and assess the claim.

Auntie Ellen came up that night after tea and took the older boys out to the pictures, to see a new innovation in the cinema. 3.D. films. Ellen was always very enthusiastic about things like that in the pictures and the theatre and the dancing, and liked to take the boys with her to the pictures and panto in the theatre, as she did not like to go on her own. She told Jim and Jackie, "its a good new film experience. You wear a pair of glasses, with a red lens o" one side and a green lens on the other, and when you look at the screen through them things come out from the screen towards you. "I don't like the sound of that" said Jackie "you night get hurt". "Don't be daft, it's only make believe pictures" said Jim. "It will be good fun". So Auntie Ellen, Jim and Jackie eat their dinner up quickly, and left for the pictures. "Thank God that get's rid of them for awhile, Ellen goes on and on and on.

No sooner had they left then Jimmy arrived home. He could sense a strained atmosphere in the house, as he washed and sat down at the table for his dinner. "What's wrong with your face?" he asked Cathie, and he could have bit his tongue, as he just remembered that the insurance assessor had been that day. Cathie placed his dinner on the table in front of him. "Enjoy your meal" she told him, "and that is for after", placing his pay-slip on the table in front of him. "Where the hell did you get that ?" and "have you been through my pockets ? You have no bloody right going through my pockets", shouted Jimmy.

"That pay-slip tells a story, and not a very pleasant one. That pay-slip was in the top pocket of your good suit, that got burnt, and it shows that you have as much for yourself as you give me to keep the house.

You're a greedy self-centred swine. You will have to put more into the housekeeping in future". She told him, Jimmy was not at all pleased at being found out, but he knew that he was in the wrong, and had to hand more money in to help Cathie with the housekeeping.

Cathie went on at Jimmy, saying, "You always have enough to buy your fags and newspapers and your drink, and to your football matches once or even twice a week. I know that I'm not the only wife to have to put up with it, there are thousands like you, I would like to change places with you, and give you the purse, and let you run the house to see how you would manage. Run the house, why, you would run away, you would not last the week. My God, my Ma was right, it's a man's world". Then again Cathie retorted, "You're a selfish swine; that's what you are". "Alright, alright". Jimmy knew that he was in the wrong, and he could not win this one; "I'll give you more money in future, don't get your knickers in a twist", he said.

"We will have to see if we can get this place back to some kind of normality, we can't live here like this with the place in this state. We will have to get the kitchen and the lobby redecorated, and see about new linoleum and carpets, once we get the insurance money through. Then there are the chairs and the rest of the furniture, not to mention the clothes that were on the pully, and the bed and all the bedding. Aye, the list goes on".

Bit John came up the stairs. They knew his heavy footsteps. He had just put his finger on the doorbell when Cathie answered the door. "Are you cycick or something ?" Big John asked her. "Never mind that, any news of Margaret ?" asked Cathie. "No news yet" was Big John's reply. "That baby does not want to come out into this world, and I can't say that I blame it", said Cathie. "They say that she might go into labour later tonight, I have to phone later to see if there is any news. How long do you think it might take ?" Big John asked Cathie. "Trust a man to ask a question like that. It's in the hands of God" said Cathie, as she told Big John to eat up the home-made soup and the tatties and ribs and cabbage that she had made. He had a big mug of tea to wash it down. "Oh' I wish that Margaret could cook like that, she's a hopeless cook. Margaret wants to be by in time to go on her holiday. With a young baby just out of hospital, if she does do it she had better be careful". "What are we talking like this for ? She's not had the baby yet". Big John then left to go and telephone the hospital, and they told him to come up as Margaret had gone into labour

"Open the envelope then Jimmy" said Cathie, "it has lain in there long enough, and lets hear what it has to say, while I get the baby fed and bathed and ready for bed, and then you can put Thomas and Frankie in the bath for me", she said. On opening the envelope he read it out to her, it was from The City of Glasgow Corporation Housing Department, and it was offering them a new home. "What a time to come, is that fate, or the work of God" said Cathie. As her mind began to wonder, she thought of a nice back and front door in Scotstoun or up in Knightswood. "Oh' they have actually offered us a house after fifteen years on the waiting list, it must have been all the doctor's lines. I'll get Ellen to look after the kids and we can go up and see them. Maybe our luck is changing at last.

Drunchapel, Drumchapel. To their horror the housing department had offered them a three apartment in Drumchapel, one of the new peripheral housing schemes. The Corporation had begun a slum clearance program to rehouse many of the tenants that were living in sub-standard housing in the old tenement building in the city centre and other parts of the city. "Go and see what it is like before we make up our minds, there is a development officer up their with keys to let you view a show flat. It would not do any harm to take a look. We will have to go home and see that the children are alright first", said Cathie..

After they had been home to check on the children, and had something to eat and a cup of tea, not forgetting a fag, they both liked a cigarette. It seemed ages before they finally reached their destination. "Thank God' said Cathie, who was glad to get off the bus. "What a long journey. We will have to find the street-avenue. There are no streets up here, they are trying to make it posh. They'll have a job, they are still trying to make other parts of the city posh", said Jimmy. Cathie replied,"my brother James said, that if anyone he knows takes a house up here, he will send them smoke signals, like the Indians to let them know that he is coming up to visit them. I think the stagecoach would be quicker than the bus. Some of the streets haven't got any pavements or street lighting yet", said Jimmy. "There's a workman, ask him for directions". "Just go away round there, cross the road, go over the spare ground, cross the road on the other side, and go all the way up the big hill, and you are nearly there. I think it is the fourth street, sorry avenue up on your left, just ask someone" replied the workman. It took them ages. "My God, imagine doing that with a pram and three kids to trail and bags full of messages, it's a nightmare" said Cathie. "You don't have to do that", "there are mobile shops, and a wee general store at the top of hill". "Aye, no competition, they will charge your what ever they like and it will be daylight robbery." "Ugh, stop your moaning, don't prejudge until you have seen the house. I would not want to walk up here in the dark after a night at the pictures, especially if it was a horror film. Look at the woods, t here could be anyone lurking behind those trees at night, just waiting to jump out on you. Oh no, give me the bright lights, and the tram-lines of Partick, anytime," said Cathie.

They finally arrived at the avenue, and half of the closes were still not finished. The large four storey building had either eight or twelve three or four apartment flats in each close. That's an awful lot of children, think of all the fighting, and trying to get your washing out in the backcourt to dry.

Brickies, slaterers and plasterers, plumbers, electricians, gas-fitters and painters there was plenty of work for tradesmen and their labourers. Cathie and Jimmy had at last arrived at the address which they had been given, and went in to view a couple of flats. Other people, mostly young couples arrived to view the flats, and they all soon got chatting, asking questions like:- "where do you come from? how many of a family do you have? what is your present house like ", all anxious to know the background of their new neighbours. Cathie remarked to Jimmy, that she thought that most of them seemed nice people, although some of them seemed a bit rough. As they continued their tour of the flats in the close and up the stairs, it became apparent that twelve three apartment flats up one close with mostly young couples meant that there would be a large amount of children up the close. Cathie liked the look of the flats. The main door opened into along narrow lobby, with a bathroom situated behind the door, and a small bedroom to the front on the opposite side of the lobby. Futher along the lobby, and on the same side as the bathroom was the kitchenette, which was very small and narrow, "unsuitable for an average size family", Jimmy commented. On the outside wall was situated a steel and glass door, leading to a small verandah, looking out onto the backcourt. Cathie was "what a daft idea, that will make it easy for people to break in". Although, she did like the two wally sinks, one which was bigger than the other and ideal for steeping clothes. She then commented to Jimmy, "Take a look out at the back-court again. How are all these families going to get a washing out with just four poles to tie the washing lines on ? You would have to get up at six in the morning, or draw lots to see who gets their washing out, and I have to do a washing every day to to keep my waines clean, and I suppose most of the other mothers will be the same". On the other side of the lobby was a drying press, and at the other end of the lobby was a larger bedroom to the back, and it had a large window and a tiled coal fire-place. Last, but by no means least, they came to the livingroom, they opened the door and entered. "It's a good size, square, and I like the long four-framed window, it lets in plenty of light" Jimmy said. "Honest to God, I cannot make a desicion, I like the flat, but I don't like the location, it is too far away from the shops and the buses", said Cathie, and continued, "if the kids are ill, how do I get to the nearest telephone, never mind the nearest doctor. Another thing", she continued, "these vans and mobile shops that come round the streets, they will charge you what they like. The alternative would be to get a bus into Clydebank or the city, and that will add to the cost of your shopping. Yes, no, I don't know, I like the house but not the place", stated Cathie. "Well, it's up to you, but I think we should take it for the sake of getting an extra room. We will need it now that we have got a girl" said Jimmy. "We will go home and sleep on it, and ask Jim what he thinks", said Cathie. "What's it got to do with him ?" asked Jimmy, and he continued, "you ask for his opinion too often if you ask me". They made their way to the bus stop, where they waited and waited for the bus to arrive. They waited, fifteen minutes, half-an-hour, forty minutes, until the bus arrived. "That's ridiculous, and there is not even a bus shelter or a shop door-way to stand in for shelter from the rain, and think what it will be like in the winter. "Just think, said Cathie, standing here with bags of messages and a couple of kids". "I will be glad to get home", said Cathie, and continued. "Our Ellen is alright watching the kids for us, but she is no use attending to them. I'll need to get them fed and ready and into bed before I can relax myself, I never seem to get a minute to myself these days.

After they had thanked Auntie Ellen, and she left to catch her tramcar home, Cathie asked Jim if he had been fighting with her again, to which he replied, "No, she would have told you if I had been, you know she has a big mouth" Jim replied. "That's enough of that, that's no way to speak about your auntie", his Mammy told him. Then as they all got ready for bed, Cathie and Jimmy asked Jim if he would like to go and see the place, but as he had already been up with his auntie he knew what it was like. As Cathie and Jimmy lay in their bed they discussed it, "weighting up the pros and cons". They only got a few hours sleep before they had to get up. When she woke up in the morning, Cathie thought that as there were no public houses in Drumchaple, it might keep Jimmy off the drink.

They decided to move. The money that they would get from the Co-op insurance along with the money, that was left out of Jimmy's accident compensation should help to furnish and get carpets, and other things that they would need to get. They agreed to flit, and put their flat up for sale. Cathie said, this hasn't been a very lucky home to us anyway, apart from getting a lovely wee daughter.

A close meeting was held for the new tenants to ballot for the new flats, and the next day Jimmy went to sign the missive and get the keys. Then it was off to view the flat again with Jim, and to meet some of their future new neighbours. Cathie and Jimmy liked most of them, who were young married couples with two or three children, just like themselves.

It would take some time to move. Margaret was still in the hospital, past her time, and with high blood pressure. Cathie had her two boys to look after along with her own children, and the two men's meals to make for them coming home from work, along with all the other household chores. Even with the burning smell from the fire, along with the sight of her lovely kitchen destroyed, she still had to cook and do the washing in it. She told old Joe "the day that we have to more can't come quick enough now", and said that she hoped that he would be alright, but he had members of his family who would go up and see if he needed anything. They could even apply to get him a home-help, he should have had one long ago. "We have put the flat up for sale, and I hope that somebody nice buys it, and pops in to see you", said Cathie. "Oh, I'll no get neighbours as good as you, still you've got to get on with your own lives, you are doing the right thing, moving away to a ground floor flat with a young family, you shouldn't be bumping a pram up four flights of stairs. The ground floor flat and a wee garden to put the wain's pram oot in will be good for you and your wains", said old Joe.

Chapter Eleven
HAPPY BEGINNING, SAD END

Two weeks past her date and Margaret gave birth to her new baby. "Mother and baby doing fine", cried out Big John as Cathie opened the front door to him. He was a bit disappointed as he told Cathie that it was another boy. "Thank God they are both alright, and the baby is like the world as your Granny would say". "Have you got a name for it, sorry him yet ?" asked Cathie. "Aye, Margaret is thinking of calling him one of these new names, Brian", replied Big John. "That is a lovely name, is to be the Godmother ?" Cathie asked. "We thought of asking May", answered John. "Good idea, she will like that. Our May is Godmother to, I don't know how many wains". "Margaret still wants us to take her holiday, with our boys and the new baby, to Fife" said Big John. "You're suppose to get a child christened first before you take them anywhere" said Cathie. "We'll manage, we have been looking forward to this holiday. I feel I really need one myself", replied Big John.

Aunties May and Ellen came up to take the children out to let Cathie and Jimmy get the packing done, well some of it for their flitting. Cathie had managed to get a lot of it done when Jimmy was at his work. Jim said "I hope you are not taking us to that graveyard again, it is making us frightened at night". "Don't be daft", said his Mammy, "the living will do you more harm than the dead", looking at Jimmy as she said it. The two aunties took the children out to Kelvingrove Park, and to visit the Art Galleries again. Jim said, "I'm never away from this place, I should have gone out with my pals". Auntie May replied "Never mind, we are coming back again after tea to take you to the pictures". Auntie Ellen interrupted, "you should be grateful that you have two such very good aunties to come up and take you out".

It was 1955, and the cinema had to compete with television, and the next night Auntie May and Auntie Ellen took the boys to the pictures to see cinemascope, the wide angle screen. Rock n' Roll films like "Jailhouse Rock" and "Rock around the clock" and singers like Elvis Presley and groups like Bill Halley and the Comets, were becoming very popular with young people. They found the music very infectious. They got up from their seats and sang and dance in the cinema, but unfortunately they would get carried away and rip out the seats and start to fight among themselves and form gangs. As the fighting continued and the manager stopped the film and the police were called in, some arrests were made.

Exciting times, Harold Mac. Millan was telling the people of the country that they "never had it so good". "You've never had it so good, It's just like a win on the football pools", said Jimmy. "What are you talking about ?" Cathie asked him. "Well the insurance money has come through, and the flat has been sold for £350, and that's £50 more than we paid for it in 1952. The flat was bought for cash just two weeks after it was put on the market. It was bought by a Scots woman who has worked in the States and wants to come back home to retire. The money from the insurance would help to buy things for the new home, although Cathie did not think they got the true value. She was delighted that her beloved tubby chairs were saved in the fire and could be recovered. Oh, Cathie loved her tubby chairs, as if they were some kind of status symbol.

Cathie and Jimmy went out on a spending spree, it was a case of spend, spend, spend when they went out to the shops and bought things for their new home. It was one of the periods of their marriage when they were really happy. If they had come up on Littlewoods Pools, they could not have been happier. They did not buy wallpaper or paint, because they had to wait for a year for the plaster to work had dried out and the final defects had been attended to.

They went up to the new house every day that they could get the children looked after, measuring this and checking that. As soon as the linoleum and the carpets had been delivered, the two of them were up laying it down, and they got tiles glued down on the kitchenette floor.

Aye, it was really beginning to look good, and Cathie was beginning to like the place. They had always fancied having wall-lights, since they had seen shell shaped wall-lights on the walls of a house that they had visited, and also in a lounge bar that they had visited up the town. So, they decided to get an electrician to come and fit them, and Jimmy would plaster up the walls. "The wall-lights will really set the livingroom off", said Cathie.

A lovely new bedroom suit was bought for the back bedroom. It also had a gents wardrobe and a lovely shaped dressing table with a big mirror. There was a large double bed with a mahogany headboard. Cathie thought that her tubby chairs would look nice in the back bedroom as it had a nice interior grate coal fire. It would be nice and cossy in the winter for getting ready for bed or to sit and read or knit and listen to the wireless, and to get away from that television for a while! Cathie was not to fond of television and thought that some of the programmes were just rubbish. But the kids loved it, and it kept them quite for a while.

Three weeks later the removal men arrived at the close entrance in their large removal van. The removal men came up the stairs. There were five of them. Two big heavy-set guys, two medium size guys and a wee bloke, and there was not a pick on him. Cathie felt sorry for him. "What could he carry ? a lamp-shade ? all the light stuff". They came in and had a good look around. One of the big heavy-set guys was still puffing and panting as he went into the front room and he shouted out to his pal. "Wully, Wully", (he sounded in a state of panic), and Wully replied "Whit's up Mick ?" Mick shouted as Wully entered the front room, "A piano, a big, a large up-right piano" Mick shouted still puffing and panting. Having another look around, they decided to get the piano down the stairs first with their ropes. "It's gawn'y be a hell o' a job gettin' that thing doon the stairs, but we'll manage it somehow" Wully the gaffer said to Cathie. Wee Jim said to Wully "Aye mister, ve've got a piano, and there is nobody in the house who can play it". His Daddy told him, "Shut-up, you've got too much to say for your own good, so you better button your lip for your own good"

At last the removal van was loaded, and the flat was empty. Cathie with the keys in her hand walked round for just one last look, and with a tear in her eye, she thought of the good times that they had in the house, and then the bad. She had a lump in her throat as she thought of her good neighbors and friends that she would be leaving behind. Some came out of their doors to say "cheerio", and to wish with them good luck in their new home, and some of them waved from their windows. But on the other hand Cathie's thoughts turned to the ground floor flat with the garden at the front, where she would be able to put the baby out in her pram, and keep an eye on her. Cathie, Jimmy and wee Jim left the house for the last time, locking the glass door and then the stormdoor, and walked down the four flights for the last time.

All the furniture and their belongings had been loaded into the van, and Jimmy got into the back with the removal van with the men, and Cathie and Jim got into the front passenger seat with the driver.

The van engine started up and the driver drove along Dumbarton Road. Cathie hoped that it might just be the start of a better life, and Jim shouted out "Good-by Partick, look-out Drumchaple, here we come".

Up Crow Road and along Great Western Road and they were up in the Drumchaple housing scheme in no time. It was a lovely hot day. The sun was shining, and the schools had just broken up for the summer holidays. There were children everywhere, playing on the street, playing in the gardens, and playing on the spare ground. There were children everywhere, hundreds of them, and you couldn't half hear from shouting and squealing.

It was just as well that Margaret had got out of the hospital with her new baby boy, Brian, the previous day. Big John had taken the two boys home, and they all went up to the hospital to get their Mammy and their new wee baby brother home. Margaret had arranged to get the baby baptised, so that she could go on her holiday, soon after she came home from hospital.

Cathie and Jim gave the van driver directions, and in no time he had found their avenue and stopped at their new close. As the van drew to a halt they noticed that a few of the windows had curtains up, as a few of the new tenants had already moved in. Jim said "I wanted to be the first up the new close". Cathie told him not to be so childish; and continued to say that she would hate to be the first tenant to inhabit the flats as it would be extremely eerie up the close, alone.

Cathie, Jim and the driver jumped out from the front of the van and the driver went round to the back to open it up to let Jimmy and the other removal men out. After having to carry the furniture down four flights of stairs, they were delighted to be told that the new home was on the ground floor. They had been dreading carrying the piano up stairs.

Cathie and Jim went straight into the house and opened the door to let the removal men bring the furniture in. Big Mick, one of the removal men, kept repeating "thank fuck", it's low down. Cathie went straight into the kitchenette to make the men a welcome cup of tea, as they places the items of furniture in each of the rooms, and then had a sit down and a smoke, and that welcome cup of tea. Then they left with a handsome tip in their hands. They got into their van to drive off, and Cathie and Jim went to the window and gave them a wave as they drove off out off the avenue.

Removal vans were coming and going all the time, bringing the furniture and belongings of the families that were still moving into the new flats. Some of the families had enough furniture to furnish a three or four apartment house, but most of the families were coming from either one room and kitchens or single-ends, and hadn't enough money to buy new furnisings. A few had the bare essentials, a bed or two, a table etc., and a couple of tea chests. Many were unemployed or low income families, who had come from tenements in the city, and had either been sitting rent free in abandoned properties, or had been paying very low rent. Many were genuinely worried about having to pay a bigger rent, or pay a rent at all, not to mention the added expense of having to buy extra curtains and linoleum and a bit of carpet.

Every day new arrivals moved into the flats, and each close was nearly full, as the workmen continued to put the finishing touches to the buildings, and the pavements and street lighting.

It was a lovely long dry hot summer in 1955 when they moved in, and they did not have to light a fire for months. Cathie did not have to worry about the children going out to play, as she could just look out of the window to see if the baby was alright in her pram in the garden at the front, and look out from the verandah off the kitchenette to keep an eye on Thomas, who was now five years old, as he played with his new little pals in the back-court, and she could hang over the verandah to break-up any fights that he got involved in. Jim, who was now twelve years old, went off to explore which was a new adventure land. Through the woods, over the road, down to the village past the Girning Gates, and down to Peel Glen to the Bluebell Woods. Sometimes he would forget the time, and it would suddenly begin to get dark, as he and his pals hurried to find their way home. Jim arrived home to a good telling off from his parents, but at the same time they were relieved to see him home safe and sound.

In the summer the only means of getting hot water for baths was to fill up the boiler in the kitchenette with water, and once it was hot enough, it had to be carried into the bathroom in big pots and emptied into the bath until there was enough water in it to have a bath.

At last, Cathie felt a lot more contented in her new home and the surroundings outside. Although it did take a bit of getting used to after growing up in a tenement near the city centre, "it's not too bad", she thought, as she stood looking out of the long livingroom window. "We still have a lot of work in front of us, and this is not going to get it done", she said to Jimmy. The curtains were up, the linoleum and carpets were down, and the furniture was in its place. They still had to put up the new bed in their room, after spending nights sleeping on the bed-setee in the livingroom, and make it up with new sheets, blankets, pillows and pillow-cases. "You know what they say about a new bed", said Jimmy. "Forget it, not tonight, or any night, if I had my way" replied Cathie. "Ah' what's the game?" asked Jimmy, by this time getting very randy. Cathie told him that if she had her way the first child would have been the last, and that the rest had been conceived by force, with him with a drink in him. "I did not want to have any more kids after the trouble that I had at Jim's birth, but, thank God the other kids are alright, and I love them, and would not part with them for the world. All I need now is a good nights sleep, and so do you by the look of you" said the very tired Cathie.

At last the tea chests were finally emptied. The last of the dishes and pots and pans and the children's toys had been found a place and put away. The bags of extra food, messages that Cathie had bought on her last visit to the Co-op in Partick, just in case she could not get a van in the morning. The thought occurred to her, imagine building all these houses for big families, and not making any provisions for shopping for the essentials, butcher, grocer, chemist, and a dairy for milk and rolls in the morning. Not forgetting the ciggies, I'll have to get plenty of my "Willy Woodbine" in, I couldn't do without a fag in the morning. A wee fag helps to calm my nerves. "I think I'd murder that man if I didn't have a fag in the morning, or when he comes in to calm my nerves", thought Cathie.

There was a general store up the hill, at least it was handy, even if they charges you what they liked, a penny on this, a half-penny on that. There was always a queue a mile long, and Jim hated going to it, because they always served the adults before the children, which was not fair because most of the children's Mammies were also in a hurry to get their messages, and could not get out because they had young babies at home. Cathie had made the porridge for the breakfast and wondered what had happened to Jim and the milk. Just then Jim arrived with the milk and the rest of the messages and a newspaper. "Good a newspaper, at least we can see what's on television tonight" he said. "Not tonight, the man is not coming up untill tomorrow to fix the aerial" replied Jimmy. "Could we not try with a coat hanger to see if that will work, and get us a picture?" asked Jim. "I wonder what kind of reception they get up here?" said Jimmy. "I don't know about reception, but there is one guarantee, and that is that the programmes will be awful, they always are" said Cathie. "Not always Mammy", said Jim. "There are quite a lot of programmes which I find interesting and entertaining" Jim continued. Cathie replied "you would be better concentrating on your homework for school, your qualifying examinations will be coming up in one years time, and you know that you have missed a lot of schooling, through no fault of your own, and you have a lot of catching up to do. So ask the teacher to give you extra homework". Jim was not too happy about that, but agreed.

The next morning they all woke up early, and the sun was shining through the windows. Cathie noticed that it was quiet, the sound of the traffic that she had got used to going along Dumbarton Road was no longer there, and for the first time in years she could hear the birds chirping and whistling, and she could smell the newness and freshness of the house. Jimmy got up and made a cup of tea, a plate of porridge and had a smoke and left for work on his bicycle. Cathie got up and let the boys sleep on in their bedroom a while longer. She got baby Kathleen bathed and fed, then dressed and put her out in her pram in the garden at the front of the house. It was then that Cathie thought that it really did make a difference not having to bump the baby's pram down four flights of stairs, and she could open the window and look out to see if she was alright, and listen to hear if she was crying.

Thomas was next to waken and get up, and he was washed and dressed and then he had his breakfast, acompied by a spoon full of cod-liver oil, which Cathie got from the clinic. Thomas hated the taste of cod-liver oil, and would screw up his face, and try to spit it out, saying, "Oh Mammy, I hate stuff, do I have to take it ?" His Mammy replied "Yes, it will make you big and strong". "Can I go out to play ?" he asked his Mammy. "Alright, as long as you stay in the garden at the front, or play in the backcourt, with your new friends from up the stairs, and stay where I can keep an eye on you. "Don't go away", remember what I have just said, "Don't go away". "O.K. Mammy" he shouted as Cathie opened the door and let him out.

Jim had a long lay-in and got up near lunch time, and went to the shop, that he hated to get his Mammy some messages. Cathie went out into the garden to bring the baby into feed her, and met her next door neighbour, whom she had met once before, when they were getting the keys for the houses. She seemed a nice friendly soul, and Cathie was sure that they would get on well. Cathie then took the baby and the boys in for something to eat and a big glass of milk. After spending some time in the house Thomas got fed-up and asked his Mammy if he could go out to play again. Cathie agreed to let him go out and repeated her earlier warning, "Thomas, play either in the backcourt, or in the garden at the front, and don't go away, stay where I can keep an eye on you".

Cathie could hear the sound of children playing in the front, and in the backcourt, when she was in the kitchenette preparing the dinner, and she assumed that Thomas was still there.

A short time later she went out just to check, and Thomas was no-where to be seen. Cathie was very worried. Thomas had wondered off with some older children. He was away for some time and Cathie became increasingly concerned about his where-abouts and safety. She asked Jim and the older children that were playing in the avenue if they would look for him, which they did. Then she asked the woman next door if she would keep an eye on the baby, which she did, and Cathie also went out to look for Thomas. As time went by, they stopped everyone that they met and gave his description and asked if they had seen him, the answer was always the same, No. Sick with worry Cathie and the children continued the search for Thomas. "I am going to dial and report him missing to the police. Where is the nearest telephone box ?" Cathie asked a woman, and the woman replied, "You'll be lucky to find a telephone box in this God forsaken place". As Cathie continued her search for her little boy, Thomas, she was about to go into the shop to ask if she could use their telephone, when Gordon, one of Thomas's pals, who stayed up the stair, and Thomas had been playing within the backcourt, came running down the road. When he saw Cathie, he began to squeal "You wee boy has falling into a swamp, and he is drowning". When poor Cathie heard this she was frantic. She asked Gordon, "quickly, take me to him, show me where he is". As Cathie and Gordon ran up the road, for about five minutes or so they were soon followed by an army of children, all eager to assist in the search. A few more yards up the road and over the hill, and Cathie's anxiety turned to joy and relief as in the distance, she could spot little fair hair boy coming up the hill towards her. Thomas spotted his Mammy, and began to run as fast as his little legs could carry him, crying loudly and into the arms of his Mammy. Cathie gave him a big hug, and then a right telling off for going away. Cathie then asked him what had happened to him, and Thomas replied, that he had just gone for a walk with his pals and fallen into the river. Cathie said that to her knowledge there were no revers in Drumchaple. The older children, who had been helping in the search informed her that it was just a burn.

Cathie took him by the hand and led him down the road home, and repeated to him the warning "Don't go and wander off again, the next time you might not be so lucky". After Cathie collected the baby from her next door neighbour, and called Jim in for tea, Cathie got Thomas stripped of his wet clothes, gave him a good wash down , and dried him and put on dry clothes. She lit the gas boiler in the kitchenette to get hot water for baths. Just then Jimmy, who had been working late, came in from work. He was in a good mood, for a change. After he had had his dinner, Cathie told him what had happened to Thomas, and then got the children bathed and into their beds. After a day like that, Cathie would have been glad to go into the livingroom, and put her feet up in front of the telly, but no such luck. After a cup of tea and a cigarette, she had to go into the kitchenette and light the boiler yet again to boil water for another big washing. She had to do a big washing every day. With twelve families up the close, and only four close poles, the women had to do their washing the night before, if they wanted to use the backcourt and hang their washing out the following morning.

Margaret and Big John had gone off on their holiday to Pittenweem and gave Cathie the address of their holiday accommodation, in case she and the family would care to go up and pay a visit. Cathie and Jimmy though that as the weather was still good, and their children did not have a holiday this summer, it would be a good idea to take them on the train up to Fife to pay a visit. The family had not had a holiday for a couple of years and it was good for the kids to get a breath of good sea air. Cathie also felt that she too needed a change of scene.

At the weekend they got the children all bathed and into their beds early, as they had an early rise in the morning to catch the train at a mainline station. Cathie and Jimmy had a bath, and an early night in bed themselves, and they were feeling very happy with the thought of going away for a wee trip. They became very passionate towards eachother and made love. They all got up early, they all got ready, had breakfast, and set off to catch the train to Fife.

After a journey of several hours they were very glad when they eventually reached their destination, and got a taxi to take them to Margaret and Big John's holiday accommodation. "I hope that they are in, I will have to feed and change Kathleen again, she's getting heavy for six months old, andI'm dying for a cup of tea and a fag" said Cathie.

The taxi took them to the address of Margaret and Big John's digs, and after paying the driver, they got out the taxi and collected their things. Cathie went over and chapped the door, "Yoo Hoo, is there anybody in ?" she shouted as she chapped the door. The door opened and Margaret and Big John called to their sons, "look who's here", Jackie and Frankie came running to the door, and were delighted to see their Auntie Cathie standing there holding the baby and their cousins. "Well don't just stand there on the door step, come in, its an awful wee single-end, you couldn't swing a cat in it. It still has a gas-mantel" said Margaret. "My God, that brings back some memories, and not very good ones either, well come of them were good" said Cathie, and she continued, "Lets have a sit down and I can change the baby, have a cup of tea and a fag and then we can take the wains to the seafront, after all that's the reason we came, to get God's good fresh air".

"Where are we all going to sleep if we stay the night, there is only one double bed ?" asked Cathie. "We'll manage, the women and the two youngest can sleep in the double bed. There are plenty of blankets, so the two men and the older boys can sleep on the floor its only for one night, they say that sleeping on the floor is supposed to be good for your back", said Margaret. "When did you start to worry about my back, after all the bags of coal that I've carried", replied Big John.

At last they were all ready to go out for a walk down to the seafront. It was a nice dry sunny day, with a bit of a cloud in the sky, and they could enjoy the sea breeze in their faces. The men played on the seafront with the boys, at football, and after a while the boys wanted to play on the swings, and the men got fed-up. They wanted to go for a pint in the pub, as usual. Cathie told them to go and said that Margaret and she would look after the children, but she warned them, "A pint or two, and don't forget the road back, as you normally do, Jimmy". So off the men went to the pub. After a wee while the women got a big cold and fed-up just sitting around, so they collected the boys from the swings and went off for a walk around the shops to buy some messages in and see if there was any bargains to take home. Cathie and Margaret then made their way back down to the seafront where they had arranged to meet their husbands, but there was no sign of them. Cathie said "That yins stuck in the pub, once he gets the taste of drink, he can'ny stop until his money runs out, or until he is pie-eyed". A few minutes later Jimmy and Big John came and met their wives as arranged and they went back to the single-end for dinner.

The only thing that they could do in the evening after they had all been fed, was to go out for another walk. Jim said "this is a boring place there is nothing to do". "Yes there is, walk, it's good for you" said his Daddy. "Yes, that's right, walk, walk, walk, who do you think I am King Billy ?" asked Jim. "That's enough of your lip. We'll take a stroll down to the chippy, and then we can nip in for a pint" said Jimmy. "That's right, think of yourself as usual" replied Cathie. "Oh get a grip, screw the heid, your no here tae fight" Big John butted in.

The men went off to the pub for a quick pint, and Jimmy had a wee chaser. "you can'ny beat a wee goldie, the water of life, as they say". "Who say ?" asked Big John. "They say, the men who make it, the distillers. Aye, that's one thing about Scotland, the best country in the World for making whisky and steel, ships and a lot of other things" said Jimmy. "That's an interesting conversation, son", said two old men sitting at the next table. Jimmy was just about to go over and join their conversation, when Big John had to remind him, "Don't forget the women and kids, or well be in the bad books, and I don't want that for the rest of the holiday, so come on Jimmy, sorry pals but it's time for us to "sling our hook", and they left eh pub to go and join their wives and children to make their way back to the single-end holiday digs. On the way back they stopped at the chippy to buy some fish and chips, although they were not very hungry, it was just something to do to pass the time on this great Scottish holiday, as boredom set in. On their way back they had to pass another pub. "No way, just keep walking" said Cathie. "Just a wee cerry-oot, for a wee night cap. After all, we are are the one's who have to sleep on the floor tonight" replied Jimmy. "As they say, it's good for your back" said Cathie. "there is nothing wrong with my back" replied Jimmy. "Just your big fat bum at the bottom of it" said Jim. "that yins getting worse, cheekier by the day" said Jimmy. "Only a joke" shouted Jim, who was beginning to get a bit worried, that he had said a bit too much.

It began to get dark and there was a slight drizzle of rain as they made their way back to the single end. As they made their way along the road Thomas shouted that he needed a wee wee, and the rest of the boys and both fathers had to go and "spend a penny" down a lane. "That's terrible" said Margaret, and BigJohn replied "men can't hold it in the same as women". "That's all the drink that you've swallowed" said Cathie. "I feel a lot better for that stated Jimmy. Big John went to the chippy to get the fish and chips, and he told the other to carry on up the road, and said that he would catch catch up on them as he was a very fast walker.

They hurried back to the single-end, and opened the door to get in, and it was very dark. It felt very eery. "Quick put on the light" cried out the boys. "Find the switch" said Jackie. "There is no switch, ya mug, it's a gas mantle" replied Jim, who continued, "Hurry-up Mammy and find the matches". Cathie found her matches and lit the gas mantle, and then the cooker and put on the kettle for a nice cup of tea to go with the fish and chips. Just then Big John arrived at the door with the fish suppers for the adults and pokes of chips for the boys. "I bought pickled onions and a bottle of tomato sauce" he said. "You know I don't like tomato sauce" said Cathie. "You can have an extra pickle then" replied Big John. They'll all got "stuck-in" and enjoyed their fish and chips, and the boys had cups of "ginger" to wash it down.

Once every had finished their fish and chips, the children and the adults were beginning to feel a little tired. "We had better get the sleeping arrangements sorted out for the night" said Margaret. "Yes, and we have got Mass in the morning, we better get up early in the morning to find out where the chapel is, it's a sin to miss Mass even on a holiday" said Cathie. "Right, let's get the bed clothes out what we can do" stated Margaret. The two Mammys slept in the big double bed in the bed-recess with the younger boys, and the two babies shared a large pram. They seemed to be settled down well for the night. However, it was a different story for the husbands and the two older boys. They spread the blankets and pillows down on the floor, and took their clothes off and slept in their underpants, and tried to settle down for he night. The floor was very hard, and they could feel a draft coming from the door. "I hope there are no mice in this house that come out at night, or even rats" said Jim. "Don't say that Jim, you'll make me scared" replied Jackie. "Shut-up, and get to sleep" was shouted at them by their Daddies. They tossed and turned for hours trying to get to sleep. They had just dosed off to sleep when Jim heard something, and then felt something. "Oh no, Oh no", he shouted at the top of his voice, "there is a mouse in here". "There is a moose loose aboot this hoose" he shouted. "It's your imagination, so get back to sleep", they all shouted at him, being angry at being woken-up.

It was a long night, but daylight eventually began to shine through the window. Everyone felt very tired with lack of sleep, but decided to get up and make the most of the day before Cathie, Jimmy and the kids left to go home.

As they were tidying up the single-end and preparing breakfast, there was a knock on the door, then another followed by a much louder knock. It was the owner of the single-end. She was very angry, a neighbor had gone round to her house to inform her that, her single-end was over-crowded, and that there were two families staying there instead of one. The owner was most upset with Big John opened the door to her, and he assured her that their visitors had only spent one night there, and were going home that day.

After Cathie and Margaret had found a chapel and had gone to mass with the children, Big John and Jimmy had gone to the hotel for another "wee swally" or the "the hair of the dog". They met up with Cathie, Margaret and the kids and went to have some lunch and another walk down to the seafront before the visitors left to make their journey home.

They all enjoyed their weekend away. Cathie thought that the children all looked good after their weekend of sea air, especially the baby, who had lovely rosy red cheeks. She also thought about the pile of dirty washing she had to face that night when she got home, or the next morning. Cathie also hoped that the shop would still be open when she hot home to get some messages in, or that there would be a van in the avenue, to get something in for Jimmy's piece for his work in the morning, and for fresh milk and bread or rolls.

Monday morning and the schools were starting back after the summer holidays. Jim was going back to the same special school, and the grey school bus was coming to pick him up at the end of the avenue. Thomas was starting school, and that morning was very exciting for him as he was going to attend the new school that had just opened in the scheme with some of his new pals.

Jim got his jacket and put his brown school cap on. Although his school did not have a uniform, Cathie liked to dress Jim in a brown blazer and school cap. He made his way along the lobby towards the outside door with Cathie who opened the door to see him off. "I hate going back to school, I wish we could always be on holiday" he said. His Mammy replied "you know you need a good education in order to get a good job when you are older, so stick in at your lessons, you know that next year you will be doing your qualifying examinations. I would like to see you passing and going to an ordinary school, with normal children". An ordinary school with ordinary children – this got Jim thinking. I must be abnormal or something. Jim asked his Mammy "what is an ordinary child ?", and his Mammy replied "You'll miss your bus if you don't hurry-up. Cheerio", and the door was closed. Jim made his way out to the corner of the avenue, where the school bus was to collect him at eight thirty, but he waited and waited.

At last Jim's grey school bus arrived, and as it stopped at the corner to pick him up, the lady attendant opened the door at the back of the bus and put the steps down to let Jim on to the bus. The children from the avenue saw Jim go onto the school bus, and began to shout, "Jim's a loony, Jim goes to the loony school". They gestured with their hands, and stuck out their tongues at the children on the school bus, not knowing that although the children on the bus had a physical handicap, there was nothing wrong with their intellect, and some of the other children were slow developers. The back door of the bus closed, and it was off to the start of a new term.

When Jim got home from school and got off the school bus at the end of the avenue, some of the children were playing at the entrance of the close. When they met Jim, they said to him, "we didn't know you went to the loony school". Jim told them that it was not a loony school, and children just went there because they had bad arms or legs, and some of the children had other handicaps, and that it was not nice to make fun of them.

He was glad to get down the path and ring the door bell. Cathie opened the door, and asked Jim how he got on at school on his first day back. "O.K." he replied, adding that he did not get much work to do. "You would like that" said Cathie, as Jim went passed her and into the livingroom. He asked Thomas how he liked his first day at school, but he, was not interested, and just replied "not bad", as he continued to play with his cowboys and Indians on the floor.

Just then the door bell rang. Cathie said, "I wonder who that could be. Jim, go and see who is there". Jim went and answered the door. He shouted out with delight, "Its Auntie Margaret and Uncle John". When Cathie heard this, her heart missed a beat, she thought it was bed news, and something was wrong. "What's wrong" she called out. "Its good news, wait until we get into the livingroom, and we will tell you", said Margaret. "Its great to see you. I've not seen you for weeks" replied Cathie. Margaret hurried into the living room and took a set of keys out of her pocket, and rattled them at the baby, who was sitting on Cathie's knee getting fed. "Hello, you blonde beauty", Margaret said to the baby as she picked her up. "So, what's your news then Margaret" asked Cathie, and all in one breath Margaret told her. "We got a letter from the housing department, which offered us a new house, and we went to see it, and these are the keys, and more good news, its just a bit up the road from you, not very far, just ten or fifteen minutes walk. I seem to follow you everywhere, and I always wanted a house in Drumchaple" said Margaret. "Yes, that's true, you do always seem to follow me everywhere" Cathie replied.

"By the way, Margaret, I think that I might be pregnant again" Cathie told her sister, adding, "its the last thing I need. I never know where I am with that man of mine. He is alright one day, and all wrong the next". "It might be your age, 41, maybe your going through the change of life" Margaret replied. "I hope your right. I don't think I could handle another kid, especially the way that that man of mine is behaving at times. Do you know he's getting very odd, and acting very strange at times, maybe its the effect of all those falls and head injuries in these accidents. I'm dreading the start of the football season, I know it began a week or two ago, but he has not been to a match yet. He'll want to go one of these Saturdays, and I'm dreading it. I get really fed-up when he goes out to a game only on a Saturday morning, and says that he will be in for his tea and never arrives home until late at night steaming drunk, or sometimes I don't see him until the following morning, with a great big hangover. But, worse than that is when he brings a stranger, and sometimes two or more back to the house on a Saturday night, and expects me go give them a meal, the soup and the meat that I have made for Sunday dinner. It takes me nearly half the day on Saturday getting the vegetables all cleaned and scrapped for the soup, the meat prepared and a trifle made, (the wains love a trifle)".

Cathie made Margaret and Big John a cup of tea and a bite to eat. They really enjoyed it because they were famished as they had been out for a very long time. After they had eaten, Margaret who was so very excited about getting a new house, said to them, "Lets take Cathie and the kids up to see the new house, and we can have another look".

"It seems to be up hill and down dale to get to it, more up hill" said Cathie. "It will be more down hill going to your house when you return" replied Big John. They reached the new buildings, which were built by a different contractor, and were of a different design from the building in which Cathie lived. The brickwork and the windows also were different. They went up the close, which had only three flats, one on each landing. "That's good, you wont have a next door neighbours to bolher about, and your stair will be a lot quieter and probably a lot easier to keep clean" said Cathie. Once inside the flat Cathie noticed that on entering the lobby, which was very narrow and long, that with the exception of the livingroom door at one end and a bedroom door at the other, all the doors where on one side. There was a window in the lobby looking out onto the backcourt. The walls were very think, and there was only one fireplace, which was in the livingroom to heat the hot water, and no fires in the bedrooms. "This will be a very cold house in the winter, how on earth are you going to keep it heated. It will get damp. You are bound to get a lot of snow and frost up here in the winter. There will also be strong winds blowing, if not gales, and you will hear them living on a corner at the top of a hill with nothing in front of you for protection, like this" said Cathie.

Margaret and Big John moved into their new flat a few weeks later after like Cathie and Jimmy, getting a quick sale for their one room and kitchen and toilet flat in Partick. It took some weeks for the money from the sale of their flat to come through. They moved in couple of weeks later, and soon got to know their new neighbours. With the money that they got after they had paid off the loan, they bought new linoleum, and a new dinning-room suite. Big John was getting plenty of overtime in the shipyard where he was now working, and was also going on ship trail, and playing football whenever he could find the time, and this was also bringing in extra money.

Margaret liked ornaments. She was always buying ornaments, but not very expensive ones, which was just as well as the children were always breaking them. When the boys broke the ornaments, she would just go out and buy new new once.

A building contractor was constructing a bloke of flats which would also contain a row of much needed shops on the ground floor, but it would be sometime before they would be ready to be occupied, so in the meantime Cathie and the rest of the housewives had to depend on the mobile shops that went round the scheme, and look out of their windows to see if the long queues were going down. If they waited too long the van would be half empty, and they would have to go to the shop at the top of the hill to stand in another long queue in order to get the rest of their messages. All this activity took up a great deal of their time.

By this time Cathie was getting to know her neighbours really well and became very good friends with some of the other mothers up the close, and they confided in each other about their families and their worries and problems, and of course woman's trouble. Jim would go to ask his Mammy something as she and a couple of the other women were standing at the close having a wee blether, and she would say "Away you go this is women's talk", and Jim replied, "I only want the key to go into the house to get something to eat, a piece 'n jam, or a biscuit, or an apple".

He would say to himself, "I don't know what these women get to talk about".

Cathie confided in Margaret that she feared the worst and added that she had better go to the doctors surgery and have a pregnancy test. She confided in Margaret that she, as she had had already had four wains, was nearly sure that she was pregnant, adding, "I don't know how that bloody man of mine will take it".

Cathie walked down to the doctors surgery in the village with baby Kathleen, (who was just six months old), in her pram after seeing the boys off to school, and wondered how she would manage with two babies, then she thought, "women who have twins have got to manage, never the less, its something that I could do without".

As she sat with the baby on her knee in the consulting room, she asked the doctor if he was sure, as he confirmed the result of the pregnancy test. She said to the doctor, "My baby's only six months old and I have my hands full with the other two, not to mention that man of mine. Are you sure doctor ?" she asked again. "I'm sure, its positive", the doctor replied. "Oh well, its another wee gift from God, and it will be loved just as much as the others" said Cathie, and she continued with one of her favourite sayings, "As long as its like the World". I don't know how that husband of mine will take it". The doctor asked, "How is he behaving himself this weather, is he keeping off the drink ?" Cathie replied, "He is off the drink at the moment Dr. Mac Nabb, but I dread the start of the football season, that's when he breaks out, if you know what I mean. He is acting a bit funny at times. I suppose all those accidents and falls on the head are bound to have some effect" she replied. Cathie left the doctors surgery and made her way up to visit Margaret to tell her the news. She felt she would have to talk to someone. Jimmy came home from his work some hours later, and after he had a wash and sat down to his dinner at the new formica table that they had just bought for the kitchenette. Cathie had put down a big plate of her home-made soup, which he loved, she put plenty of vegetables into it and also oat meal, and it was so thick that you could almost stand on it.

When he had almost finished his meal, Cathie sat down at the other side of the table. "I have got something to tell you. Remember that night of passion ?" "Aye, what about it, do you want another one ?" he replied. "You'll be bloody lucky. Well, I'm pregnant again, and its something that we could have done without. I was at the doctors for a pregnancy test and I'm going to have another baby" she told him. To her surprise he was delighted, and said "I hope its another girl, and we will have a gentleman's family, two boys and two girls. I really hope that it's a girl". "You take what God gives you, and as long as it's like the world and I'm alright, I'll be happy. I still have the other three to rear" Cathie replied.

"I will have to buy you a new washing machine. I saw them advertised in the Daily Records", said Jimmy. "No, I won't be the talk of the steamie", said Cathie. "They don't have a steamie here, they don't need one with two wally sinks. Ugh, you know best" replied Jimmy. After a little time thinking about it, Cathie agreed to let him buy her a washing machine. She thought to herself, "If he dose not go out and buy me a new washing machine, he will only go out and drink the money, and spend it on his boozy pals, and he only sees them when he has got money to spend on drink. "Alright, I agree" said Cathie, "we can go to the electrical shop at the weekend and see what they have got. Then again, we might need the money for other things with a new baby on the way". Jimmy would not take no for an answer.

They got up quite early on Saturday morning, got the bus into town and had a good look around the electrical showrooms. After looking at all the various makes, they decided to purchase a Parnal, which had an electric ringer. "That will be great, no more kawing the ringer handle, the other modles that they saw still had a ringer handle that you had to "kaw". "Since it is a Saturday morning and we are out this far, we may as well go and have a look round the other shops, and go and see what's on offer the Barra's, sometimes you get a really good bargain".

A week later, on the Monday morning, wash day, after Jimmy had left for work, and the boys for school, the delivery van arrived at the foot of the path. The men carried the washing machine to the entrance of the close. The neighbours were at their windows or stood at the close entrance. "Is that something new your getting ?" they asked Cathie, who felt almost guilty telling them that it was a new washing machine. "A washing machine, have you come up on Littlewoods, have you won the pools ?", the neighbours asked Cathie.

The delivery men dumped it in the middle of the kitchenette, which was so very narrow. Cissy from next door came in. "Come on in Cissy, you can help me take this packing off and I'll have a read at the instructions"

Cathie called out to her. Cathie was a we bit frightened of electricity, but knew how to put on a plug. "They have not included a plug. How is it that when you buy something and pay a lot of money for it, they can't include a plug ?" stated Cathie. "You'll no get a plug anywhere in this place", replied Cissy. "I'll just have to take one off the iron and put it onto the washing machine and we can try it. I'm frightened of these new fangled gadgets" Cathie said. "Aye, I hope it doesn't blow the hoose up, wae us in it" replied Cissy. Cathie fitted the plug, and wondered if she had wired it correctly. "I hope I don't blow a fuse, I don't think I have any fuse wire in the house". "How is it that when you put things in a safe place, you can't find them when you need them. I'm still not organized since I came here. I have other things on my mind". Cathie told Cissy that she was pregnant. "Don't worry I'll be here to help you when the time comes". Cathie was a wee bit relieved to hear that, as she was worried what would happen to her children when her time to go into labour came.

Once the machine was filled with water from the sink tap by means of a rubber hose, Cathie added Tide soap powder, but there wasn't enough in the packet. So she had to send Cissy up to the shop for another packet, and she came back with Persil. Cathie poured it into the water in the machine and stood back, and with trembling hands switched it on. A wee red light came on, then she puched the handle to start the agitator, and it moved, round to the left, round to the right. "Stop" shouted Cissy, "you have forgotten to put in the washing". "Silly me", said Cathie as she put in a pile of dirty clothes and started up the agitater and the clothes began to wash. The door bell rang and Cathie hurried down the lobby to open the door. It was Serah, another neighbour. "Ah'm just in to see how you are getting on. What's that noice ?" she asked. She was just in to do her "nosey parker". "Oh my God, Cathie, what's that coming from your kitchenette ?" Cathie turned around to see soapy suds coming out of the kitchenette, she had put too much soap powder into the washing machine. Chug chug chug came the noise from the machine as the soapy foam came out over the side and onto the floor. Cathie ran in and stopped the machine, and they began to clean up the mess. "At least the place will be clean – and damp. I'll need to dry it out". At least the washing was nice and clean and Cathie put it through the electric ringer and into the sink. Then she looked out of the kitchenette window to see if there was room left on the washing line to put the washing out to dry, but the line was full, so she had to put the clothes upon the pully.

After they had got the place all cleaned up, Cathie asked Serha if she would like to have her washing done. "Oh, yes please if you don't mind" Serha replied, then she went into her house and brought a pile of dirty washing in. Cathie put it into the machine, with not so much soap powder this time. Serha was delighted and said that it would have taken her half the day to get that lot done. She kept repeating these words as she took her washing into her house to hang up on the pully, and said "I'll be able to put my feet up for a while before I get on with the rest of my housework. Cathie said "I'd better get on with my own housework. I have a lot of catching up to do, and I'll need to go and get something in for the dinner, it's never ending, who said that a woman's work is never done".

All the neighbours up the close were really getting to know one-another and were beginning to have parties in each others houses on special occasions, like childrens birthday parties and the New Year.

The football season had begun several weeks ago. "I don't mind you going to the match. I know that you like to see your beloved Thistle. As long as you come home for your tea and sober. I don't mind you having a pint, but you can't stop at a pint, you have got to get "pie-eyed" and want to fight, and make the wains and me upset. Why can't you come home in a reasonable manner ?" asked Cathie. Jimmy replied 'I won't get drunk, and to prove it I'll take Thomas with me to the game, and that will keep me out of the pub". "That's good" said Cathie, for she knew that Thomas was his favourite, and he would not like anything to happen to him. So she got Thomas ready, and though to herself "he will watch him like a hawk". As they were leaving the house, Cathie saw them to the door, and she warned Jimmy "guard him with your life, if you let anything happen to him...and don't forget no drink and come straight home". About an hour after they had gone, Jim was sitting at the table at the livingroom window, trying to catch up with some homework for school for Monday. He looked out of the window and saw Auntie Ellen coming. Cathie went to open the door to her, and as she did Ellen was standing there all dolled up, with brightly coloured clothes, big dangling earrings and the make-up caked on. In her hand she had a big message bag. Cathie took her into the livingroom and said, "you're looking very smart, where are you getting all the money ?" Ellen replied "mind you're own bloody buissness, it's my buissness what I do with my money". Then she turned nice because she was up for a favour. Cathie made her tea and something to eat, then she asked Ellen why she had the big message bag with her.

Ellen always knew that Cathie always kept a large stocked coal bunkerker out in the close, an that she could always reply on Cathie' simpathy, and understanding, said explained that she could not get any coal in her street, as there were never any coalmen going around the streets of Scotstoun. Poor old Granda can't keep warm in his bed even with his big wally hot water bottle and loads of blankets and quilts". "But, it's still British summer timeEllen" Cathie reminded her. Ellen replied "the weather can turn cold, especially at night". So Cathie gave her some coal in the bag, and then Ellen left to go and visit her other sister, Margaret, and she repeated these visits often during the winter.

Jim put on the television at teatime when children's hour was on. It was a puppet show called "Whirlygig" with Mr. Turnip. He did not like it, but sat there and watched it anyway. Cathie made the dinner and fed the baby, and looked at the clock, and began to worry. The time was going on and Jimmy and Thomas should have been back from the football match. Jim and she had their dinner and it was getting near the end of "The Six-Five Special". Jim loved the show, introduced by Josephine Douglas and Pete Murray, and introducing Rock n' Roll singers like Nancy Whiskey, Lonnie Donegan, Cliff Richard and many, many more.

Cathie was still watching the clock with the programme had finished and it was beginning to get dark. There was still non sign of Jimmy and wee Thomas. "If anything has happened to my wee boy I will..." thought Cathie. Just at that minute she heard Jimmy's key going into the lock and they came in. Thomas came running up the lobby, all excited. He was followed by his Daddy, who kind of staggered behind him. "You've been drinking" Cathie said to him. "I have not" replied Jimmy. "I can smell the drink off you, and you are staggering. You are an irresponsible swine, you can't be trusted with wains, you make me sick". Cathie was annoyed. Jimmy did not answer her because he knew that she was right, and as Thomas was his favourite, he would not have forgiven himself if anything had happened to the child. Cathie questioned Thomas for information about what had happened when they were on their way home from the football match. To her anger, Thomas told her that his

Daddy had left him in a swing park on his own, and went to the pub. He continued to inform his Mammy, "it was beginning to get dark and I was the only one left in the swing park, and I was hungry and dry, and I wanted to go to the toilet. I was getting very frightened and was beginning to cry when my Daddy came and I did a wee wee, and he brought me home. Cathie was incensed when she heard this, and a big fight broke out. There were many angry words spoken, and the verbal abuse continued for some considerable time. One thing led to another and it was beginning to get a bit out of control as they began to throw things at each other. The children got very up-set and began to cry, as Jim tried to defuse the situation. When Cathie realized this she stopped shouting, but Jimmy continued uncontrollably until Jim pushed him into a bedroom and closed the door, hoping that he would go to bed and fall asleep. Everyone went to bed, Cathie in the children's room.

During the night the baby, who had a cot in the boys room began to cry, and they could not pacify her. Jimmy was awakened by the sound of the baby crying, and came running down the lobby and burst into the room to see what had happened. He was standing there with a string vest and no underpants on, and he had the string vest pulled down to hide his private parts. They told him to go back to bed, and as he turned around to leave, they could see his big bare bottom. As he left the room he said something very odd, very odd indeed, Jim thought; Jimmy said "There was a man under the bath", yes very odd indeed.

The months passed quite quickly. One morning after she had seen Jimmy off to his work. The boys were away off to school, and she had fed and bathed the baby. She was doing her housework, and she knew the signs. She knew that she was going into labour. She could feel that her waters were going to break, but she did not panic. She took baby Kathleen into Cissy her next door neighbor and asked her to look after the baby, and also if she would go and telephone and ask if the doctor or a district nurse or a midwife would come. This Cissy did at once, she was only too glad to help, and her own children were away at school.

In the meantime Cathie had everything prepared in the back bedroom for the delivery of her baby. The doctor and the midwife arrived to see that everything was in order. The midwife stayed with Cathie, and the doctor said that he would return to see who her labour was progressing.

As the pains of labour began Cathie prayed to Our Lord, Our Blessed Lady, and the Saints that she and her baby would be alright.

As the day dragged on Cissy took Kathleen in her buggy to the shop and to collect Thomas from school with her own children. After returning and getting the children organised in her house, She got Meg another neighbour to look after the children while she went to see how Cathie was getting on. The midwife was still in attendance, and as it was winter, there was a big coal fire in the grate, but Cathie, was well on in her labour, and was feeling the heat and they had to open the window to let her cool down.

Cissy went back into her own house to give the children a meal, while waiting for Jim's school bus to arrive at the corner of the avenue. A short while later the school bus arrived and Cissy called Jim into her house. She told him that his Mammy was in bed ill, but did not tell him why, no one told him what was happening, and he was worried. Unusually for him, he did not feel like eating, and did not finish his meal. He repeatedly asked what was wrong with his Mammy. No one would tell him.

Some hours later Jimmy returned home from his work, and went in to see how Cathie was getting on, then came in to see the children and have a bite to eat and a cup of tea, before returning to his own home to see if Cathie was ready to give birth. He did not go back into the bedroom, as he thought that a place of birth was no place for a man. He sat in the livingroom waiting for news. Cissy's husband, Pat returned home from work, and was chatting to his own children and Cathie's boys. The midwife went into the livingroom to inform Jimmy that he had a lovely new baby daughter, and that mother and child were both well. The words that every father loved to hear about his wife and new born child. Jimmy rushed into the room to give Cathie and the very small baby girl, with brown straggly hair a kiss. Then he went into the next door neighbours to announce that the children had a new wee baby sister.

The two boys rushed into their own home as excited as could be. Jimmy carried Kathleen, who was only thirteen months, and still only a baby herself, and did not know what was happening. Hurriedly they went into the bedroom, and were very pleased to see their Mammy. As they sat on top of the bed she showed them there new wee baby sister, who was asleep in Kathleen's pram by the side of the bed. "A baby, that's a baby in my pram" was all that Kathleen would say. "We are going to call your new wee baby sister Patricia" Cathie told them. "That's a nice name. Where did she come from ?" asked the boys. "She's a gift form God" replied their Mammy. "In that case Mammy, does that mean that we came from Hell and are a gift from the devil, because Mammy you always say that we are wee devils", said Thomas, and Jim butted in, "and he (his Daddy) is always telling me to go to Hell". Cathie replied "Don't you start any trouble, Jim, this is supposed to be a happy time for the family".

After a night's sleep, interrupted by the two o'clock feed, and up again at six in the morning, Cathie was up the next day doing her normal housework and looking after the children. The midwife and health visitor made a visit to see Cathie and the baby. They nearly had a fit when they saw that Cathie was up so soon after giving birth, and doing all her normal work. Cathie told them that there was no one else to do it. Everyone had their own children and homes to look after, adding that her own mother had a large family and had to manage.

Margaret came down later and went to get the shopping in. She said that she would take the boys up to her house after school to let Cathie get a rest.

Chapter Twelve
"Jittery"

Margaret was asked to stand for (to be Godmother to the new child at the Christening) of the new Baby. She was delighted to accept. The new baby was christened the next Sunday at the priest's house in the village. He used the garage as a makeshift chapel. But there was no party in Cathie's house afterwards as money was beginning to get tight, and people didn't seem to bother much about having christening parties after the first child. This time Jimmy did not bother about which religion the child would be baptised into. Both he and Big John were working that Sunday, and they would not miss out on a chance to work overtime, as it was paid at double time rate.

Miss Docherty told the class that this was a very important year for their education. They were preparing for the qualification examination, and that she would be giving them a lot of homework: mathematics, English, history and geography, and the children would have to study very hard, especially Jim, who had miss quite a substantial amount of his education through having to attend clinics. She gave him quite a lot of hamework, but did not correct it for days.

The class was still going for cookery lessons, and Jim and his pals enjoyed baking fruit cake, baked apple, lemon merangue pie and the home-made soup, but their favourite was the delicious fruit cake. Jim and his pals loved to take that home to let their Mammies taste it, but they had most of it eaten on the school bus before they reached home.

Jim had a very nervous laugh, and the least wee thing set him off. Once he started to laugh, he could not stop, and people would get angry with him and tell him to stop laughing, the more harder it would be for him to stop, much to the annoyance of the teachers and his parents. Miss Williams, the big fat grumpy cookery teacher bent down to take some cakes, which the class had made, out from the oven, and as she bent down, she let off (broke wind) and Jim began to laugh, saying to Wee Pat his pall who was standing next to him "Its no just the cakes that I can smell", and he began to laugh. Miss Williams turned around and told them to stop laughing, and by this time the whole class was laughing. Miss Williams singled Jim out as the instigator. She then marched him down the corridor, past all the classrooms and up to the headmistress's office. The teacher knocked on the door and was called in by the headmistress. Miss Williams told her what had happened, (or her side of the story, and leaving out that she farted, thought Jim wait until I get a chance to tell my side of the story...she farted), but he never got a chance to get around to that. Miss Dow, the Headmistress, went on about insulting a non-Catholic Englishwoman, and gave Jim six of the belt, three strokes on each hand. It was the worst belting Jim had ever experienced. His hands began to sting as he left her room and as he walked down the corridor, he blew on his hands to try to take the soreness of the sting of the belt away. He felt like crying, and the tears were beginning to come from his eyes. "I'll take it like a man", he said to himself as he wiped the tears away with the end of his sleeve. He went back to the class and did not say a word for the rest of the lesson, and his three pals, all called Pat, were all anxious to know how he got on.

New baby Patricia had celebrated her first birthday. She was a very small girl, with straight brown hair, and was very smart for her age. Her big sister, Kathleen, who was just one year older, and her two big brothers, Jim and Thomas, who were now twelve and six years of age, helped to bring her on, and this made her old fashioned for her age, as people would say about her. Before she was a year old she could walk and talk, and could run about the house. The other children would laugh as they all sat watching the television in the evening and wee Patricia would go up to the screen and talk tot he people on the programmes. "Aye, she was a right wee comic".

The day of Jim's qualification examinations was the following morning, and he went to do some studying in preparation for the test. Cathie told him that he had to go to bed early, and get a good nights sleep. Jim woke up during the night and he could not get back to sleep. He tossed and turned, trying everything that he knew to try and get back to sleep, then he said a decade of the rosary, he counted sheep, he folded his arms to try and keep them from shaking, but the harder he tried to keep them from shaking the more they would shake. After a couple of hours, he managed to fall asleep. His worst nightmare happened in the morning. Jimmy had forgotten to set the alarm clock the previous night and they had all slept in. Jimmy was late for his work, and said that he would be locked out, and said that he would go in at lunch-time. Jim was ill with worry, and cried out "What am I going to do, how will I get to school, I've missed the school bus, and I will be late for the start of the qualification examination. What am I going to do ?" "You will just have to go down the road and get a corporation bus to school, but be very careful" said Cathie. "You would think that I have never been on a bus before on my own the way you are going on. I'll never make it and the buses are bloody hopeless, about one every half hour , if they come" stated Jim, who by this time was extremely flustered.

Jim went to the bus stop and waited, and waited and kept looking at his wrist watch. At last a bus arrived at the shop and he go ton and paid his fare and took a seat. As the bus continued on its journey it stopped at every stop on the route, and Jim grew more anxious by the minute. He could feel himself breaking out into a sweat and his hands begin to shake, and his face begin to twitch as the time went on.

At last after a horrible time on the journey, the bus reached Jim's destination, and he was glad to get off. He made his way through the streets of Anderston as fast as his wee legs could carry him. Running through the main shopping area, He met Auntie Mary, who was out doing her shopping. "What are you doing here ? Where are you going ?" she cried out to him. "I'm late, I'm late", he sounded like the rabbit going to the tea party in Alice in Wonderland, and wished that he was at that moment in time. "I've got to get to school as fast as I can", he shouted to her as he ran as last as his legs could carry him, falling a couple of time, scraping his hand and his knee, but he was sued to that, he just got up and carried on.

After arriving at the school entrance, he went in and dashed along the corridor, only to be shouted at (stop running boy) by one of the teachers, (if she only knew) thought Jim.

Jim made his way through the school as fast and as quietly as he could, and up the back staircase to the classroom where the examination was just about to begin. Trembling with nerves and feeling a wee bit squeamish, he stumbled into the classroom. "What happened to you Jim ?" enquired the teacher, and she continued, "You have just made it in time, you can tell me later. Have you brought your ball point pen, you know that no one came read your hand writing if you use a nib pen". Jim's hands were still shaking as the "qually" (qualification examination) began. As he began to write his hands began to get shakier, the ball point pen became wet and slippy as Jim's hands began to sweat and the paper got wet as the nervous perspiration dripped from his head onto the paper. This worried him, and it was sometime, and a couple of papers later before he could concentrate, but by this time he was in despair, as he knew in his own mind, that he had not reached his full potential.

Once the results of the qualification examinations were known and the parents of the children had been notified. Cathie arranged a visit to the school to see the teacher, and discuss the implications of the results regarding Jim's future education. Miss Doughtery thanked Cathie for coming to the school to see her, especially as she knew that she had three younger children to attend to. Cathie had told her that Jimmy was on night-shift that week, so she had left the children with him. "I was very dissapionted with Jim's marks and performance. I thought that he would have achieved a higher grade. He has been a changed boy lately", said the teacher, and went on to tell Cathie about the incident with the cookery teacher and the headmistress. She added that she had found it" out of character for Jim to behave like that". When Cathie and Miss Doughtery saw the headmistress in her office they found her perturbed. Cathie explained to the teacher that Jim had been experiencing a difficult time at home, and added that this had probably reflected in his behaviour at school. When the headmistress heard the explanation, she agreed that if a doctor found Jim medicinally attainable, then he could start attending an "ordinary" secondary school at the start of the next term.

When Jim arrived home from school later that day, Cathie was waiting for him. He rang the door bell, and his Mammy opened the door, but, before he was halfway up the lobby, Cathie gave him a belt round the lug. "What was that for ? What have I supposed to have done ?" he enquired. "You know only too well, and don't act the innocent with me", said his Mammy. Continuing, "giving up cheek to the cookery teacher and the headmistress, and they said that if the doctor agrees, you can attend a secondary school" said his Mammy. Jim, however, had mixed feelings about this. He was pleased about the prospect of attending a school with so called "normal" children, but, on the other hand he was afraid of the children not accepting him. But at least it was getting near the end the term and there was the summer holidays to look forward to and that would take his mind off it for awhile. The examinations behind them, ment a more relaxed period in the class until the end of term. Most of the school work was done in the mornings, and for an hour or so in the afternoon of each day Miss Dougherty read one of her favourite books "Anne of Greengables" the teacher would get carried away with the story and read on and on, and the children enjoyed listening to it. Sometimes Miss Doughtery would ask some of the children in the class to read a paragraph or two if her voice began to fade as her throat dried up, but the children really enjoyed it, even the boys, some of them thought that it was better than doing work.

The cookery lessons continued, with the usual home-made soup, apple dumplings and fruit cake etc. One day Peter, one of Jim's pals made a remark about the teachers posterior. Jim could feel himself begin to laugh again, and he knew that he would be in deep trouble. However hard he tried – he held his breath, he tried biting his lips – however hard he tried, a big laugh just came busting out. Jim though to himself, "I'm in for it this time, I'm a dead man. I'm really for it, it's that wee buggers fault, that wee Peter, it's him who made me laugh". Miss Black turned around, "You again" she shouted at Jim, and before he had a chance to open his mouth to explain, Miss Black got hold of Jim's ear and pulled him out of the class and all the way down the corridor to the headmistress's office, Jim thinking to himself, "that bloomin old witch is going to pull my ear off". When they arrived at the headmistress's office and knocked on the door, the door opened and Miss Black practically threw Jim in. The old headmistress grabbed hold of him and pushed him into a chair by her desk. She turned on her desk lamp and it shone into his eyes, (it was like a gestapo interrogation). She really lost her temper and got hold of his hair and pulled it back, and again threatened to stop him going to a normal school, and again Jim received four strokes of the strap, two on each hand. His hand really began to sting as he left her room and walked down the corridor, but at least it did stop his hands from shaking for a few minutes, as they tingled with the pain of the belt.

By the time that he got home Jim was really ill with worry. He repeated to himself, "What am I going to tell my Mammy, and what is he (his Daddy) going to say, will it result in another belting ?" He was shaking like a leaf by the time that he got off the school bus and arrived at the door of his home. He nervously rang the door bell and his Mammy opened the door, (Cathie could read him like a book, and she knew that something was wrong). "Tell me what has happened Jim. I know that there is something wrong". Jim told her his side of the story and Cathie went up to the school the following morning and everything was sorted out. Jim was allowed to go to the secondary school after he had enjoyed his summer holiday.

It was a Saturday morning and they all had a bit of a lie-in. Cathie got up and did all her usual chores, made the breakfast, got the children washed and fed and went out to get the weekend shopping in. Then she told Jimmy that if he was not going out, he could look after the younger children, and that she would go to the Barras and take Jim for company. She wanted to buy new clothes for the children, and that Jim could help her carry the parcels. She said that she wanted to get new rig-outs for the two wee girls, and dress them identically. Jimmy agreed to look after the younger children. So after Cathie and Jim had got the groceries, they set off to get a bus into town to go to the Barras. Jim loved the atmosphere as they walked around the stalls looking at the goods on sale. He listened to the Glasgow "patter" being spoken and shouted by the stall holders, as they tried to attract the crowds of people. The place was getting really busy, it was jam-packed with people with message bags, and Jim held on to his Mammy's hand in case they got separated in the crowds and he would get lost. His hand slipped from his Mammy's grasp, and Jim feared that they were about to get separated in the crowds. He managed to get hold of the tail of his Mammy's coat and was holding on as tight as he could as they were pushed along with the crowd of people up and down the narrow passages between the stalls. Jim looked up every now and again as he heard the stall-holders shouting out to there prospective customers, "Come and get a bargain of a lifetime" or "You'll never be able to buy it cheaper anywhere else in Glasgow". Cathie said, "Don't dilly dally, Jim. I want to get what I came here for and get home as quick as I can. I don't like leaving the younger children too long, even if it is with your Daddy".

They had been out for what seemed ages , and Jim said to his Mammy, "I'm fed-up, and I want to go home. You are not going to get what you came for, you don't seem to like anything that you see, Mammy". A few yards further down the passage in the main market in the Barras, Cathie saw a stall selling children's clothes. She went over to have a good look; "Oh Jim, they have got just what I am looking for, for your two wee sisters". Jim was not really interested. He was more interested in the records on sale on the next stall, and looking at a list of the top twenty, to see which record was at the top of the charts. Cathie looked at the children's clothes. There were beautiful dresses and coats and hats to match. Aye, Cathie was spoiled for choice, she did not know what to buy, and asked Jim his opinion. "Don't ask me,, I'm a boy, I don't know, it's what you like" he replied. Cathie chose identical red and white coats and hats and lovely frilly dresses for the two sisters. Chathie was so pleased with her purchases, she told Jim that it was the boys turn to get something new next. Jim said to his Mammy, "What about yourself, you have not bought anything new for yourself for ages". "Don't worry about me, we'll go to a cafe and get a cup of Bovril before we go and get the bus home. The buses will be packed at this time on a Saturday, and if we don't hurry we will meet the crowds coming home from the football matches" Cathie told him.

"Standing room only", shouted the conductor as he came to collect the fares. It was a long "shuggle" to Drumchaple from the city center, especially if you had to stand. Nobody got off the bus until it reached the housing scheme, but plenty of people got on, and they were like sardines packed into a tin. The passengers were pushing and shoving to get past as the bus reached their destination. When Cathie and Jim reached their destination, they made their way down the passage of the blue bus, and got off at their stop. To his horror, Jim felt as if death was about to strike him; "Mammy !" he called out, "where is the parcel that I had on the bus ? I had the string around my wrist. I still have the string but the parcel has gone". "Oh my God, what are we going to do" she said. They both felt ill. "We've got Kathleen's parcel, but not wee Patricia's. They were in turmoil. They did not know what to do. Should they go home with one parcel, or should they wait and see, if by chance the bus came back on that route and still had the parcel on it. They waited for the bus to return, and they inquired from the conductor if a parcel containing a wee girls dress, coat and hat had been found and handed in. No such luck. They made their way home in despair. They could have cried as they made their way down the hill to the close. Jim kept telling his Mammy that it was all his fault, and that he should have been more careful, and how sorry he was. Cathie told him that they could try the lost property on Monday morning, and that there was a good chance that it would have been handed in. This gave him some hope and cheered him up a little.

They went into the house in despair, and Jimmy said "What's wrong with your faces ?" as they went in the door. "Cathie told him what had happened. Jim thought that he was in for a belting again, as Jimmy said, "That bloody eegit; That Jim, I should have known that he would have something to do with it". Cathie said, "I'll try the lost property on Monday morning and see if it has been handed in, you never know it might have been in". "You will be lucky to see it again" replied Jimmy. "If I don't get it, I will just have to go and buy her another one. We will just have to do without something else". she replied. "Aye, whatever you say, but I'll tell you this , Cathie, I've had enough of being stuck in here all day with these wains, so I'm going out for a couple of pints", said Jimmy. "There is not a pub for miles, and the buses are few and far-between, and its raining" said Cathie,trying to persuade him to stay in, for after the day that she had had , she could do without him going out for a drink, and coming back home plastered, and God knows what kind of mood he would be in when he returned. She could not persuade him to stay in though, and he left.

After Jimmy left the house to go for his pint, Cathie thought to herself, "That will probably be the last I'll see of him tonight. He had overtime last week at his work, two nights late, and a Sunday, and a Sunday is double-time. So he has got extra money in his pocket to spend on drink, although he gave me a bit extra for the housekeeping, he will have as much to himself. I'll never see his pay-packet unless something happens again, God forbid". Cathie got on with her work, the usual routine for Saturday night, get the wains bathed and into bed, boil the meat for a big pot of soup, and prepare the vegetables, not forgetting to boil the pot of peas. "A woman's work is never done", Cathie said to Jim as she asked him to get the ironing board out for her as she had a pile of ironing to do. Her only pleasure in life was a wee cigarette. She had forgotten to buy herself a packet, with all the worry about the parcel containing Patricia's clothes. "Jim", she shouted, "take the money out of my purse and see if the shop is still open and get me a packet of ten Woodbine. Get a bottle of ginger for you and Thomas and bars of Five Boys chocolate for your wee sisters". Jim took the money out of the purse and made his way up the hill to the shop, to find that it had just closed. He was very dissapointed. He looked all around him as he went down the hill, looking in every avenue that he passed to see if he could see an icecream van, but to no avail. He went home and told hi mammy that they were "out of luck", the shop had just closed and there was not an icecream van in the area. Cathie liked her lips and puffed her breath as she stood at the ironing-board. "I wish that I had a fag to calm my nerves after the day that I've had, they help to calm my nerves", she said to Jim, who replied, "I'll never smoke when I'm grown-up, it's a dirty habit, and I don't even like touching them, when you have friends in, and you ask me to pass them a cigarette". "Oh Jim, would you go and ask a neighbour if she could lend me some until the morning ? Ask Mrs Jones, she has always got plenty", Cathie asked him. "I hate going and asking neighbours for a lone of things", stated Jim. "I hate asking for a lone of things too, but in this God forsaken place, it's all that you can do until they build more shops, and that wont be for a long time", replied Cathie. Jim was just about to go on his quest when he heard the bells, bells, no it isn't the church bells, we don't have one yet; It wasn't the school bells, or the Hogmanay bells, that was a long way off... it was the bells of the icecream van. "Gods Good, I'll get my Woodin and you can get what ever you want", said Cathie. "Aye, your right Mammy, God is good. He has saved us from going up to ask Mrs. Jones" replied Jim. Jim went out to the icecream van and bought the goodies for the children and the "Wee Willy Woodbine" for his Mammy, who lit up a fag as soon as she got the packet.

Cathie and Jim then settled down to view some Saturday night television. A short time later Cathie fell asleep in her chair, and Jim dozed off as he lay on the fireside rug on the floor. An hour or so later Cathie awoke to find the fire in the hearth almost out, and the television transmittion finished. There was just a flickering on the screen and a buzzing sound. She got up and switched off the set, and nearly fell over Jim, who was still asleep on the fireside rug.

"Right Jim, its well past your bedtime, you better go to bed and get a good nights sleep, you can get a bath tomorrow night for school, and don't worry about the parcel, these things happen", said Cathie. So Jim rubbed his eyes, went off to the bathroom to clean his teeth, after being reminded, and then went into bed beside Thomas, who had made the bed nice and warm.

"He's got a drink in him, when he's not in at this time, he's wandered off with one of his boozy pals, that will be him away for the night", Cathie thought to herself as she had one last tidy-up, and a look at the clock before going off to her own bed. As Cathie lay in bed saying her prayers, she asked God not to let Jimmy come home in a fighting mood, to waken and frighten the children. Then she got up to have one last check on the babies, then went back to bed and fell fast asleep.

At around two in the morning, unknown to Cathie, Jimmy came home and he was "pie-eyed". He was accompanied by his pal, Shug and his dog. Jimmy and wee Shug crept into the house and, without wakening Cathie went into the children's room and got into the bottom of the boys bed, along with "Black Bob" as they had named the dog. It was a stray that they had found wondering about in the rain. It was absolutely soaking wet, as were the two men. The dog made a noise as it walked all around the bedroom, before finding a place to lay by the side of the bed, banging its head and body against the side of the bed as it lay down. Jimmy and his wee pal Shug got into the bed with the boys, and between the smell of drink coming from the two men and the smell coming from wee Shug's feet, (he couldn't have had a bath for about a month) not to mention "Black Bob" (the big farting dug) who kept "letting off" as he lay on the floor by the side of the bed, awakened Jim. He was feeling sick with the smell, "This room doesn't half pong", he said to himself, and was about to get up from bed until he noticed the big black dog by the side of the bed. He was afraid to get up in case the dog attacked him, and by this time his Daddy and his pal were laying in a drunken sleep. He was very much afraid. Jim lay there awake for hour after hour, and was glad to see daybreak.

The following morning when they all arouse there was a very uneasy atmosphere about the house. Cathie got up to prepare breakfast and get the children ready for Mass. She was ready to tell Jimmy just what he could do with himself and his Big Black Bob. She spotted Wee Shug, who was a complete stranger to her coming out of the children's room. "Who are you ?" Cathie enquired. "Oh, that's wee Shug, ma pal", said Jimmy. Sensing a hostile atmosphere, wee Shug said that he would "have tae get doon the road". "Nice tae have meet you hen" he said to Cathie as he made for the door. "Wait a wee minute, have you not forgotten something ?" Cathie asked him. "Naw hen" Shug replied. "What about Black Bob here ?" Cathie asked him. "He's no mine hen, he belongs tae Jimmy, its your mans' big dug. Ah've never seen it in ma life before. See you again sometime hen. Cheerio the noo", he said. as he went out and closed the door, leaving them with the dog. "We'll just have to keep him" said Jimmy. "That will be right, I'm taking the kids to Mass, and it had better be away by the time I return" said Cathie. "It's hard enough trying to run a house, feed and clothe the kids with the money you give me from your wages, without the extra cost of having to feed that big thing. Get rid of it, and another thing, who would look after it all day while you are at your work ? Do you not think that I have enough to do with two young children in a pram to look after, without trailing a big thing like that by the side ?" said Cathie.

When Cathie and the children returned from church, Jimmy and Big Black Bob had gone. "I wish that bloody man would go to Hong Kong, and give me some peace" thought Cathie.

The last day of term, and Jim had mixed feelings about leaving his special primary school for spastics and children with other handicaps. In one respect he would be sorry about leaving some of his wee pals that he would not see again, and some of the teachers and staff whom he liked, but in another respect, he would be glad to see the back of some of them, and he thought to himself, "That's life".

Miss Doughtery was retiring, and a lot of the children that were leaving were going to different schools in other parts of the city. Jim was not sorry to be seeing the headmistress and the cookery teacher for the last time, as he thought that they had given him a hard time of it, and treated him most unfairly. At the end of the last day of term he had his last ride home in the wee grey school bus, which dropped him off at the end of the avenue, for the last time. He felt quite sad as he said "Cheerio" to the other Miss Doughtery, the school bus attendant and the children.

As he went into the house he was still feeling sad about leaving his old school. Cathie asked her son what was wrong as he looked very sad and worried, and he told her of his feelings and worries about attending the new school. She told him to forget school and enjoy the summer holidays which he did, as they had a holiday in Angus to look forward to.

The family went on a two week holiday, the last fortnight in August. It was a working holiday for Cathie, as she had to wash and iron all the clothes and put them into the big trunk along with piles of soft white nappies for the baby. It was an never-ending process of washing them and putting them into the trunk, then having to take them out to use, then wash then and put them in again. It seemed to be never-ending, and a lot of hard work for Cathie.

Jim and Thomas were very excited about going on holiday. "You would think that you had not been on holiday before" Cathie told Jim. But he was just so relieved to be going away somewhere, anywhere to distract his mind from the thought of starting a new school, and what made matters worse for him was the fact that he would be starting two weeks after the other boys, because of their late holiday.

Instead of coming straight home from his work on the Friday that he stopped for his holiday, Jimmy went to the pub for a drink and was late in getting home for his dinner.

On the morning of their holiday departure, there was a big argument because Jimmy had stayed out late the previous evening and left Cathie to do all the work, the children, the final packing and making up packed lunches for the train journey. As they continued to argue, one thing led to another, and a lot of old family arguments were reopened. Then Cathie noticed that the children, especially the boys and Jim in particular was very upset. "Stop" cried out Cathie. "This is the kids holiday and we don't want to spoil it for them, so go and phone a taxi to come and take us to the station" she asked Jimmy. Before he left to telephone for the taxi Cathie told him, "We are on holiday and we are going to make the best of it for the children's sakes. We can't spoil it for them, the boys have been looking forward to it for a long time. The taxi arrived and took them to the station to catch their train. Thomas was very excited as he looked out of the window. Wee Kathleen and Patricia, the baby, slept most of the way. This time the spent their holiday in part of a lovely big house, where they had two bedrooms and a kitchen and use of the bathroom.

In the afternoons Cathie and Jimmy spent most of their time on the beach or the sea-front, until it began to rain or got too cold to sit around. The sea air tired the children and gave them a good appetite. It helped to get them down to bed early, and let Cathie put her feet up for an hour or two, before looking out the clothes that she would put on them the next day. Jimmy usually went out for a pint on his own. Cathie made sure that he had only enough money on him for a pint or two, as she did not want "a showing-up" in front of the landlady, who was still staying in another part of the house. All they did was go for long walks in the wet wind (it rained on most of the days) along the shore and coastal roads of the east coast of Scotland.

When the holiday was over they were all glad to get home, even Jim, who missed the telly! Thomas had got the football bug after he had played football with Jim and his Daddy on the sea-front, and always wanted to go out to play with the boys in the street. His Daddy wanted him to support Partick Thistle, but Cathie and his pals supported Celtic, so Thomas became a great follower of Celtic, and said that when he was older he wanted to play for them. Jimmy was not pleased at this and told Cathie that she was turning his favourite son against his favourite football team. Thomas asked Jim "Why do you not go out to play football anymore?" Jim told him that it was because the boys were beginning to laugh at the way he ran, and that they called him names when he went to kick the ball and missed. He said that it was alright for him playing in the playground, where most of the boys were like himself, and no one seemed to mind if you missed a pass or a penalty kick, or what should have been an easy goal. "Uch, it's only a game anyway" said Jim.

"Well, that's it, the school holidays are over, and its back to the old routine" Cathie remarked. Cathie felt that she needed another holiday to get over the one that she had just returned from. She still had the same old routine, cooking, washing and ironing, and she had missed her washing machine, she had got quite used to just throwing in the washing, filling it with water, adding soap powder, and switching on. Not quite the same old routine for Jim, though, a new routine that filled him with apprehension. He did not sleep much on the Sunday night, and into Monday morning. He "tossed and turned" and said his prayers over and over again, and counted sheep. Daylight arrived at last, and he felt shattered after only having a couple of hours sleep. He wished that he could lie in and forget all about going to a new school. His Mammy shouted to him to get up, after his daddy had gone off to work. Thomas was going back to his primary school down the hill, and went off to meet his cousin, Frankie, who was in the same class. Frankie's big brother Jackie was attending another primary school in the housing scheme. By this time, Jim was well on his way on the bus to his new school.

After she had seen her husband off to work for the day, "Oh! it is just great to get rid of that man during the day, and get the house to myself, "peace", and I know where he is and he won't come in drunk, not on a Monday, because he's skint !" Cathie thought to herself. Margaret came down to visit Cathie. They visited each other most mornings after they had got their housework done, and they took the babies for a walk in their prams if the weather was dry. This morning, Margaret was looking forward to going down to hear all about Cathie's holiday, and if Jimmy, "that man of yours" as Margaret called him, had behaved himself, and "stayed off the booze".

Jim was very nervous as he arrived at the entrance of his new school. The other pupils had begun attending at the start of the term, two weeks earlier, and would have the added advantage of having got to know their form teachers and their subject teachers, and had been allocated all their books.

When Jim arrived at the school entrance he was shaking more than usual, he did not know what to do with his shaking hands. He would get into trouble if he put them in his pockets, and he could not walk about with themn folded all day. He had another worry as the school secretary escorted him up the stairs to the headmasters office – how will the teachers be able to read by shaky handwriting ? Miss Kelly seemed a pleasant woman, but the atmosphere changed from one of relief to one of tension as Jim entered the headmasters office. A big dour-faced looking man, who was sitting behind his desk, continued with is paperwork, and looked over his glasses. He got up opened the door and called a prefect to escort Jim to his form class. Once in the class the form teacher introduced himself. "I'm Mr. King", Jim thought that he could smell drink off him, as Mr. King showed him to his desk.. He introduced Jim to his new class-mates, introducing some of them by name. Jim was asked to take his seat, and had a good look around him, noticing that there were no girls in the class. Then he remembered that it was an all boys school, and he knew that he would miss the girls from his old school.

Jim recognized two of the boys from his old school, and was glad to see the familiar faces. Some of the boys in the class looked like wee Glasgow hard men, and liked to think that they were. Most were dressed in denims and leather, or imitation leather jackets, and had their hair combed back in the teddy-boy style with plenty of "Brylcream" on it. Some of their jackets had studs on the back and arms, and they wore big heavy boots, which they used to kick in fights in the playground.

The teachers were mostly male. They kept their straps over their shoulders, or under their jackets. They got great pleasure in using their straps, any time, any place, any where in the school, even in the dining room when the children were having their lunch. The strap was a deterrent to some of the boys, who would be close to tears after they had got hit on the hand or both hands at once, twice or even three times, with great force by the men teachers. Some of the wee hardmen liked to show off when they got the strap by walking down the passage, their shoulders swinging from side to side, and blowing in their hands to take the sting from the strap. Once the strap had been administered some of the wee hardmen, through would be close to tears as they walked back to their seats.

Most of the boys in the school were quite friendly towards Jim. Others, though because of his cerebral-palsy, were very hostile. Jim breaded going to the dining-room because it was self-service and this was an ordeal for Jim having to carry his own plate to the table. It was alright if the meal was solid food, but if it was a meal consisting of soup or custard, sometimes he would spill it, and some of the boys would laugh at him, and others would just say "what's wrong with him ?" and the more they looked the shakier Jim's hands became. The on duty teacher or one of the dinner ladies often went up to him, took the plate from him and put it down on one of the tables. Jim would sit down then and proceed to eat his lunch. Some of the boys would tease Jim and start to call him names, saying, "What's wrong with you ? Twitchy Face", or "Why are you shaking", and Jim replied, "I can't, and what's it got to do with you ? Shut your face and don't annoy me". His big pal, James, said to Jim, "Right you, I'll see you in the playground", and James was a big fat lump, he would have made two of Jim, Jim said, "I don't want to fight", knowing that he would get into trouble with the headmaster, and also that big fat James would "batter the hell out of him", but Jim was not scared, just terrified! "Are you scared of me?" big fat James asked Jim, who replied, "No, I just don't want any trouble".

Down in the playground Wee Pete and Big Fat James still wanted to fight, saying to Jim, "Right, Twitchy Face, come on and we will have a square go, or are you feart ?" "Bugger off, and give me peace" replied Jim, who went into the playground toilets. The stench of cigarettes from the pupils smoking nearly made Jim sick, as boys were standing about smoking roll-up cigarettes and doughts (cigarette ends). The smell was disgusting, but a couple of big boys, who were standing in as corner telling jokes and talking about sex told them to leave Jim alone. Just then the school bell rang and all the boys ran out of the toilet and across the playground to join the rest of the class, who had to form a straight line in front of their form teachers. They marched into the school building and proceeded up the stairs to the form class, where the teacher checked the register to see if all the pupils were still in attendance, before they went off to different classes. A few of the boys liked to dog school (play truant), especially Mario. God knows what he got up to, but they were always in some kind of trouble. They always seemed to have money, and no-body knew where they got it from.

Jim liked the art class, making clay pots and painting. He felt that it gave his shaking hands something to do, although he did not think that his paintings were any good. However, he liked painting abstract pictures, and was into modern art. Just drawing lines and shapes, the art teacher was impressed by his efforts. "Not bad, not bad at all with your shaking hands", and Jim was quite pleased with some recognition for his effort. One day the school chaplain, Father Cook visited the art class to view the exhibits which the boys had produced, and he looked at Jim's clay pot. "You didn't make that Jim". "Yes I did Father" Jim told him. "No you didn't Jim" "Yes I did". It was beginning to sound like a pantomime, thought Jim. Then Jim's clay pot was put up on the shelf with a card with his name on it. "There you are Father, that proves that it's my work" said Jim.

During the history lesson the teacher had to leave the class and the boys who were entering puberty began to discuss sex, and what they thought they knew about it. One boy stood up and displayed his erect penis to the class, and the rest of the boys' eyes almost popped out of their heads. Then there was a noise coming from the back row of the class, it was a boy masturbating. The rest of the boys stared in disbelief. The door of the class opened and the teacher walked in. Order was restored before the teacher had time to realize what had been going on. That was an extra lesson the boys received that day, as sex education was not on the time-table. One of the boys went and reported the incident to the teacher, who in return reported it to the headmaster, who came up to the class and gave all the boys a good telling off, but he never mentioned sex.

Jim had to travel on the school bus, which was a coach on hire from a local coach company. Along with the driver a woman attendant was also on board to look after the children, and try to keep the peace, which was a difficult job to do with fifty to sixty boys on board.

As the coach was a single-decker three boys had to share a double seat, and it was very cramped. It was just Jim's luck, or the lack of it, that he had to share the same seat as B. F. J. (Big Fat James) and his wee trouble maker pal, Wee Pete. He liked to start trouble, and could not fight his own battles, and had to get his big pal to fight them for him. On the journey home from the school to the scheme Jim was sitting at the window and B.F.J. was sitting at the passage side of the double seat, with wee (small fry) Pete in the middle. Wee Pete got up and sat on Jim's knee, and Jim pushed him off; onto Jim's knee again went Wee Pete, and Jim pushed him off again. This continued through-out the journey. Angry words were exchanged and this hostility went on for the rest of the week unknown to the attendant, Mrs. Mac.Phee. By the end of the week Jim had had enough. Big Fat James was always challenging "Twitchy Face" to a fight on the spare ground after they got off the bus. B.F.J. said to Jim "You can't talk right, you can't walk right, and you are dead scared of me. You are older than me, but I'm bigger than you, and Ahy, I'll gee you a right doing". Jim hated the idea and he knew that he would never get any peace unless he accepted the challenge, which he did with apprehension.

The coach dropped them off at the spare ground at the corner of the road which led up to the avenues. There was a lot of shouting and name calling. Jim and B.F.J. took their jackets off and the punches began to fly as a bigger crowd of boys and girls gathered around. Jim was taking a "right doing as they say in Glasgow, "he's getting hammered, right, left and centered", and he had a cut lip. He was very glad when two workmen came over and stopped the fight, and gave them a right telling off, asking them what school they attended. Jim worried that the headmaster would get to know, and that man put the "Fear of God" in him. Jim was relieved that the fight had been stopped, because he knew that he had not "a hope in Hell" of beating B.F.J.

When Cathie opened the door to Jim she was shocked to find Jim in such a terrible mess, covered in mud, with rolling on the ground, and blood coming from his cut lip. "What has happened to you, how did you manage to get in that state, you have been fighting, haven't you, come here till I hit you". said Cathie. "Come here for you to hit me, do you no think I've been hit enough" replied Jim. "What happened anyway ?" asked Cathie. Jim told her but he begged her not to go to the school, or tell his Daddy as that would only make matters worse. "Well away in and get washed and changed and we will have our tea. He's working late", his Mammy told him. "Thank goodness for that, we'll get peace to watch the telly, is there anything good on tonight ? "asked Jim, and he continued "By the way, I hear that there is a new station starting up, "Channel Ten" and it will have adverts on it. Can we get it or do you need another know on the television" asked Jim. "We need other things in the house before that, we'll see how the money goes, your Da's working overtime just now" replied Cathie. "Is there anything wrong with him, he is acting funny at times" said Jim.

The following Monday the talk coming home on the school coach was of television programmes that they were going to watch that night, and one of the boys said that "Panorama" was going to show the birth of a baby, and they were going to watch it.

Jim settled down to look at the programmes for the evening on the television. Cathie went for a night out to the pictures with Margaret, and May, a pal, (an awfy nice wee soul) to see a horror film. "You don't need to go to the pictures to see a horror, you've got one at home" said Jim under his breath, referring to his Daddy. There was great tension in

the house between Jimmy and Jim. The younger children had been put
to their beds, and they were sound asleep as Jimmy and Jim settled down
to view the television. Jim was looking forward to seeing Panorama, and
seeing the birth of a child. His Daddy said "Right you, bed" and Jim
replied that he did not want to go to bed as it was far too early. Jim was
forced to his bed under great protestation. Jim went into his bed having
a verbal punch-up with his Daddy, who came into the room and put his
hands round Jim's neck. Jim thought that he was about to be strangled, he
thought that his hour had come. Then suddenly Jimmy pulled his hands
away, as if God had stopped him there and then from doing something
that he would regret for the rest of his life. He pulled his hands away and
ran out of the room, and Jim put his head under the blankets and also
under the pillow, and relived what had happened over and over again in
his head. He decided to tell no one, not even his Manny, because he was
scared that it would cause more trouble.

The official opening of the new chapel was a big day for the folk who
lived in the scheme. Both Catholic and non Catholic enjoyed the big
event, as it brightened up their dull lives. There was not much to do in
the scheme, no pubs or clubs, or shop windows to go and see, just sit in
and watch television, if they were lucky enough to have a set. The day the
church opened the Scottish Catholic Hierarchy walked in a procession
through the crowds into the church. It was a nice day, and the ice cream
vans "made a bomb". The Mass was by ticket only, with no children.

The following Sunday morning Cathie was up bright and early as
usual, with all the children's clothes washed and ironed, and laid out
ready for the children to wear. Off up the hill with the two baby girls in
the pram and each of her boys by her side. Cathie was up at the chapel
early, for the ten o'clock Mass and the sacraments, it was a chance to get
out of the house and socialise, and make new friends.

A few months later the parish priest announced that he was holding
a parish mission for three weeks. The first for the women, the second for
the menfolk and the third week for the teenagers. Cathie told Jim that as
he was thirteen he would have to attend. He did not like the idea much,
but after the second evening he began to enjoy the service along with the
talks from the mission priests. It was also a good excuse to get out of the
house at night, and to see some of the girls who lived up the stairs, and
have a chat to them. Jim spent a lot of time in the bathroom or bedroom

standing at the mirror combing his hair making sure that he covered the bald patch which was made by the forceps that cracked his skull at birth, the hair had never grow on that spot.

He looked in the bathroom mirror, and said a few words, and watched his mouth twitch. He remembered what Auntie Ellen had said and he said to himself, "I wish this bloody thing would go away. I hate being a bloody spastic", but he knew that it never would and that he would have to accept the fact, and make the best of life. "Life has challenges for everyone, and you have just got to do your best, and you never know what you can do until you try". Jim made up his mind to try anything that he was asked to do, and if he could do things, good, and if he could not do something, to be honest and say that he could not manage it. He got ready and went to the mission at the chapel, and listened as they sang the hymn "God is good", and Jim thought to himself, "If God is good, why the bloody hell did he let this happen to me", and he realized that night that life was going to be a struggle, he had to accept every challenge, and have the ability to laugh at himself. The priest said "what you suffer in this world you don't suffer in the next"."Now that's what I call Heaven" thought Jim. Once Jim and a couple of pals came out from the mission service in the chapel, they found a chance to chat-up some girls as they walked down the road. Jim fancied this girl, Pauline, who lived up the stair, but she didn't really fancy him, although she did speak to him. That was as far as it went, but Jim thought he would love to give her a kiss, and ask her to go for a walk, or to the pictures on a Saturday afternoon, but he did not have the courage to ask. "What was that about challenge ?" he asked himself. "Maybe the next time. My day will come".

Margaret got a job on the twilight shift at the local biscuit factory. A lot of women from the scheme worked on the twilight shift. It gave them the chance to make some extra money to buy things for their new homes, as most of them had come from one room and kitchens, or even single-ends in the city, and they had moved into three, four or even five apartments. They needed the extra furniture and floor coverings, linoleum and curtains. Margaret and her pal May enjoyed getting out of the house for a few hours each evening and away from their men and wains. They got a laugh telling dirty jokes and making the young foreman embarrassed with the sexy remark's which he received from the women. Big Issa shouted to him, "Haw, Sammy, whit's that you've goot in yur pocket, is somebody in fur a hard time o' it tonite ?" Cathie looked after Margaret's children until Big John came in on his way home from his work to collect them and take them home. The children loved it when Margaret came home with bags of broken biscuits and sand a wee song, "Beattie's Biscuits are the best, in your belly they digest, in the toilet they go west, we love Beattie's Biscuits".

Chapter Thirteen
Troubled Minds

Cathie, Margaret and May had often enjoyed a night out at the pictures now and again. But nowadays they had to travel by bus into Bearsden to go to the Rio Cinema, which was the nearest to the scheme. The bus timetable was not very reliable, and sometimes the bus would be late in arriving at their stop, causing them to miss the beginning of the film. This caused them to worry as they sat watching the film that they would miss the bus home and they would have to walk the long dreary country roads. On this occasion the three women had been to see a horror film. It was very frightening and the three woman had to walk part of the way home after they got off the bus. They felt that there was someone following them, and as they stopped to look round they saw a man in a long black coat, and as they stopped he stopped and "flashed". The women screamed and ran as fast as they could, they glanced round again to see the man disappear behind a wall, on and on they hurried until they had to separate and make their own way home, all of them very frightened.

Cathie had to walk further to get home, and she had to walk down a quiet long road with a wood on one side. It was very eery, and she was very frightened after what they had gone through. she was extremely relieved when she arrived at her own close, got to the door, put the key into the lock and turned it. She walked up the long dark lobby and opened the living room door to find Jimmy sitting in the fireside chair behind the door. He frightened her. The living room as almost dark, with just the dim light coming from a wee table-lamp in the corner. There was hardly a sound coming from the television, he had the volume turned down. Cathie could sense an uneasy atmosphere in the house, and she asked Jimmy, "Have you two, you and Jim been arguing again ?" He did not answer. "Have you two been fighting ?" Cathie enquired again. "He is in his bed sleeping," was all that Jimmy would say.

Jimmy told Cathie that Patricia had been sick again. "It must have been something she ate". Cathie always worried about her children, especially wee Patricia, who was born premature. Unlike her sister Kathleen, who was never "up nor down", Patricia seamed to take every illness that was going. Cathie said that if she was in the morning she would take her down to the doctors surgery in the village in the morning. After an examination the doctor gave Cathie a prescription, and the doctor asked Cathie how she was keeping herself, and enquired about the rest of the family. Cathie put the prescription into the chemist in the village, but they were closing for lunch. Cathie would have to return to collect it in the afternoon. It was very dull in the afternoon, and began to rain very heavily. There was no transport down to the village, and it was a long walk pushing a pram in the heavy rain. Cathie asked Margaret if she would go down to the chemist to collect the prescription before she went to her work in the biscuit factory. Margaret brought back the prescription for Patricia, and Cathie gave her some, hoping and praying that it would help her. She loved to sit and watch her two wee girls play together, there were only fourteen months between them, and they played well together.

Jim and Jackie, Thomas and Frankie loved the broken biscuits which Margaret brought home from the biscuit factory, especially the Eaton Sandwiches and Butter Puffs, which she bought and brought home on her pay day.

It was the opinion of some people that the city fathers and the planners had torn the heart out of the City of Glasgow, and that instead of building out in many of the peripheral housing schemes some of the tenement buildings in the city could, and should have been renovated and refurbished. As there were only houses in the schemes, and no places of entertainment of pubs or sporting clubs, the inhabitants of the schemes had nowhere to go, and nothing to do except stay in and watch television, or travel into the city or surrounding towns. The churches had youth activities and youth clubs started; the Boy Scots, Girl Guids, Cubs and Brownies and the Boys Brigade. The children and youth joined in large numbers, as they were glad to get out of the house, and have somewhere to go. Jim went along and joined the Boy Scots, Cathie and Jimmy insisted, and although Jim was not so keen on going as he knew some of the boys, he went along to keep the peace. Jim became friendly with some of the boys, actually enjoyed himself, and looked forward to his night out each week, playing games and singing. After a few weeks the scout leader began to teach the boys how to tie different knots with string and rope. He asked each boy to go out and sit in the middle of the circle on the floor and tie their knots, and when it came to Jim's turn he went out to the middle of the circle. He sat on the floor, took the rope into his hands and tried to tie a knot, and his hands began to shake. The harder he tried to tie the knot the shakier his hands became, and the boys began to laugh. Jim began to sweat with embarrassment, he wanted to go home and fast, then he thought fight it, make the most of it, fight it, so he tried again. The more the boys scouts laughed the shakier Jim's hands became. At the end of the group meeting, as the boys left the school, as like many other things, a scout hall had not been built. Big Wully, Wee Chick and some of their mates followed Jim down the road. They were having a jest at his handicap, making their hands shake. Andy and Pat, Jim's pals told Jim not to take any notice of them, and that they; would get fed-up and go away. "They're daft, they don't know how they will end up themselves." Big Andy shouted out loud, so that they would hear him, and "bugger off". Pat called out, "let's challenge the pigs". Jim knew from experience that they would just go on and on and the more up-set they saw him getting, the more enjoyment they would get from annoying him. Jim said to Andy and Pat "Just leave it, let it rest". He knew from experience, that if the other boys saw him getting annoyed they would continue the name calling for days, weeks or months. He hurried down the road, and was glad to get home. When he got home Cathie and Jimmy asked him how he had got on at the scouts. "I'm not going back" stated Jim. "What do you mean, your not going back ?" asked his Daddy. "Just wait I said, I am not going back, because I don't like it, and you can't make me go" replied Jim. Jim did not like to tell them the real reason that he did not want to return to the boy scouts. "Aye, you are going back" said his Daddy. "It will make a man of you" his father continued. "Were you in the scouts ? Did you join when you were young ?" enquired Jim. "That's besides the point" shouted Jimmy who was getting angrier. "Just leave it." said Cathie, who by this time had had enough. "You will waken the kids, after I have tried so hard, and for so long to get them down to sleep". "You always make excuses for him" Jimmy shouted at Cathie. "See what you have started now", Jimmy shouted after Jim as he went to his bed, his head was in a turmoil, as he thought to himself, "Maybe I should have told them the reason why I don't want to attend".

Jim just stayed in the house in the evenings after school, reading and listening to the radio in the back room. He tried to hear all the new records on Radio Luxembourg, when the reception was good and he could hear the new Rock n' Roll and Skiffle songs like "Rock around the clock" by Bill Haley and the Comets; "Jailhouse Rock" by Elvis Presley, and records by many others, including Lonnie Donnegan, Cliff Richard, Nancy Whiskey. "Does your chewing gum lose its flavour on the bedpost over night" was the favourite with the younger children, especially Thomas, who liked to sing it at the top of his voice.

One night Jimmy came home from work. He had been working late and had cycled home. It was a cold dark night, and it was raining very heavily. He came into the house soaking wet, and left his bicycle propped up against the lobby wall, and the rainwater was dripping from it on to the floor. Cathie told him to go and get dried off and she would get his dinner on the table. "Nice home-made soup, and a nice big fry-up. Do you want it on the table in the kitchenette, or do you want it in the living room, where you can have it by the fire where you can get a heat, and watch television ?" Cathie asked him. "Don't put it out just yet. I have a book to return to the library, it is over-due. It should have been returned yesterday" Jimmy replied. He was most insistent that he had to return the book that evening, and off he went with the book under his arm, and as he went Cathie shouted after him, "I'll put your dinner in the over to keep it hot until you get back", and off he went.

After an hour Jimmy had not returned from the library, and Cathie went into the kitchenette to turn off the gas in the over. She though to herself, "That bugger has met someone and gone off to the pub, but then, it's Thursday night and he is skint – the day before pay-day". As the hours went by Cathie began to get a little worried, as she thought that he had sounded and acted a bit strangely. There was something not just right, not just normal, (well, as normal as could be) about him. He sounded a bit funny in a strange sort of way. "Well, that's it! He is probably laying drunk in one of his pal's houses". Cathie tidied up the house, settled the fire, and got the children's clothes ready for school in the morning before going to her own bed. As she lay in bed trying to get to sleep, she had a strange feeling that something was not quite right. She thought of Jimmys insistence on going to the library before taking his dinner. He was always hungry when he came home from his work, and could not wait to have his evening meal served to him.

He did not return from his work the following evening, and Cathie, having no money in her purse, as it was the end of the week. Her purse was empty, and the children had to be fed, she still had some food in the house, but she could not keep fresh food in the house as there was no refrigerator. Cathie sent Jim up to Margaret, as Big John also has his wages on a Friday. So Jim went up and told Margaret of Cathie's financial problem. Margaret was very up-set about the way Jimmy was treating Cathie, so she gave Jim a loan of £5 to take down to Cathie to get the weekend messages in. Wee Patricia was ill again and Cathie could not take her out, and she could not leave the children in the house on their own. She wrote out a shopping list and gave it, along with the £5 note, to Jim to take up to the shops to get the groceries in for the weekend. Jim went up the hill to the shops and stopped to talk to some pals. When he arrived at the shop he discovered that he had lost the fiver. He was ill. He looked in every pocket, he walked up and down the road looking everywhere, on the pavement, by the side of the kerb, on the road. It was nowhere to be seen. Jim's stomach turned over and over. "I'm for it, she'll bloody murder me. What am I going to do ?" he kept repeating to himself. He went down the road, up the path, into the close and got to the door. His hands began to shake more than usual as he rang the door bell. His Mammy opened the door, "Where are the messages Jim ?" asked Cathie. "I, I, I've lost the money." Jim stuttered out. "You've what ?" shouted Cathie. Jim repeated, "I've lost the money". Wallop! he got Cathie's hand across his face, she was at the end of her tether with worry and despair. There was still no news of Jimmy, and wee Patricia was still ill. "You look after the children Jim, and I'll go and look for the money, and I'll phone for the doctor to come and see Patricia" said Cathie. There was no sign of the lost £5, but she managed to find a telephone that was working, to phone the doctor to come and see Patricia. The doctor came and saw Patricia and gave Cathie another prescription for another bottle of medicine. "Try this, and see if it helps her" the doctor said. Cathie had to go and get a loan of another £5 from Margaret, to go and get food for her family for the weekend, and get Patricia's prescription.

Cathie came back with the groceries and Patricia's prescription, and by the end of the day, Wee Patricia had improved. On the following day she was well enough to play with Kathleen.

Monday, and there was still no sign of Jimmy. Cathie was increasingly concerned. She informed the police and reported him missing. The days passed, the weeks passed and the months passed and there there was no word of Jimmy. Cathie feared the worst, and wrote to his family in England, and the missing persons agencies. The big problem for Cathie was money, or the lack of it. How to keep a roof over her head, feed and clothe her children? How would she pay the rent, the gas and electricity? Poor Cathie. Life was becoming a nightmare. She hated doing it, but for the first time in her life she had to go to the Society Security. Jim accompanied her as they went to the Social Security office. They were frightened as they sat in the waiting area along with the genuine cases. There was a selection of "wino's" and "down and outs", poor sauls who had perhaps fallen on hard times, or lost their way in life. Cathie and Jim were frightened as the sat waiting for hour after hour to be called. Cathie felt like a criminal at the questions that she was asked by the young girl interviewer, followed by a male, who was a most unpleasant person. The questions that he asked Cathie made her cry, and Jim became very upset, and felt so sorry for his Mammy, for he was old enough to know what she had been through. He tried not to let his Mammy see that he was up-set. They grilled poor Cathie, question after question. After spending hours in the office they gave her the meagre sun of £7 to keep her family for a week.

Cathie felt so rejected as she and Jim left the office, and Jim could see the tears running down her cheeks. "Try not to worry Mammy" he told her. "It's alright, son", she replied as she put the money into her purse. They walked down the road feeling very dejected and got a tramcar to Granda's house. Cathie knew that he could not help her financially. She needed someone to talk to, as she went in Cathie went in and began to cry. "Oh Da, how am I going to feed and clothe my kids on this", and showed him what she received. "I only wish that I could help you, Cathie, but I'm only a pensioner, and we find it hard to make ends meet", he told her. "I know Da, I'm not looking for money from you, I'll manage somehow, I just needed someone to talk to. I can't stop for a cup of tea or anything to eat as we have left the other children with Margaret to be looked after." Cathie told him, and they went to get a bus home.

Some weeks later a registered letter arrived with a Hong Kong post mark and stamps. As soon as Cathie opened the door to the postman who asked her to sign for the recorded delivery, she saw the writing on the envelope and recognised it was Jimmy's. Cathie thought to herself "I often hoped that that bloody man would go to Hong Kong, and give me peace. He has actually gone". Cathie went into the living room and sat down on the fireside chair and opened the envelope. Out popped a letter with bank notes. "It's from your Daddy. He's in Hong Kong", Cathie cried out. "That's a long way to go to change a library took, was it in Chinese? Is he away, (for how long). Do you get the joke Mammy? say it quickly Mammy and it sounds like Chinese", all in one breath Jim said, "How much money has he sent, can we get the television converted?" "Don't keep going on about that" replied Cathie. Cathie went up to Margaret's house to tell her that she had received a letter from Jimmy and he was in Hong Kong. "You must be joking, Cathie. You always said that you wished that that bloody man would go to Hong Kong. Your wish has been granted". said Margaret. "Yes, that's right, and I also received a payment book from the merchant navy! I am so relieved that Jimmy is alright, and that I don't have to go back to that dreaded social security office again. Also it will be great not having to worry about him coming home drunk, and bringing his drunken pals home and expecting me to feed them my Sunday dinner on a Saturday night and wakening up the children from their sleep" said Cathie. Margaret asked, "But, why did he join the Navy ?" to which Cathir relied, "God knows, I can never understand anything that he dose now. Maybe, he has gone back to his time at sea during the War!"

Cathie and her children were happy and contented with the money coming in by post. "It is wonderful with my Daddy away", said Jim. With the extra money she received (she recieved more than she got from Jimmy when he was at home) she managed to save some and buy more wall-paper and paint to decorate the house. She did the decorating in the evening after she had got the children bathed and put into their beds. Sometimes she would stay up half the night to finish a wall or a room, or finish painting a door or a skirting board or a window frame or ceiling. When it was all finished Cathie's house was looking really nice, bright and fresh and clean looking. After the cold days of winter had passed, Jim got out the bulbs and plants that Jimmy had put away the previous year, and replanted them in the garden at the front of the building. When summer arrived they had lovely blooms in the front garden, and everyone in the avenue would stop and admire the flowers and congratulate Jim on his work, and this pleased him, and enhanced his confidence.

Everyone had to get a television, it was 1957 and screens were getting bigger, going from 12inch. to 14inches to 17inches, bigger and better! All the boys in school and out in the avenue were boasting to Jim about having two television channels to choose from, the B.B.C. and Scottish Television from the Theatre Royal in Glasgow. Jim was jealous when his pals spoke of the good programmes that they saw. The adventures of Robin Hood, William Tell, The Jack Jackson Show and Cool for Cats. They all hurried home at lunch time to see a locally produced show "The One o'Clock Gang". Instead of singing street songs and songs about their football teams, the children began to go along the street and in the playgrounds of schools singing television commercials like "Murry mints, Murry mints, too good to hurry mints, don't make haste until you taste the hint of mint in Murry mints". Cathie told Jim that the needed a lot more important things for the house before television conversion.

Cathie always took her children down to visit Granda and Aunties May and Ellen after Mass on Sunday. Jim and Thomas and their two little sisters liked to go down to see their Granda and their Aunties, as it gave the boys an opportunity to take their wee sisters to the swing park. Sometimes Margaret and her children would also pay a visit on the Sunday afternoon, and they would all have a good time. Auntie May, who still worked all week in the printers made the Sunday dinner and they all enjoyed the meal before returning home.

One Wednesday evening, Cathie's door bell rang when it was quite late. Cathie did not like opening her door late a night unless she knew who was at the door. She shouted, "Who sis there ?" and the answer from behind the door was, "It's me, Ellen, open up". Cathie opened the door, and before she had a chance to speak, Ellen shouted, "It's ma Da, deid (dead)". There was Ellen all dressed up in bright colours , and looking like a Christmas tree, with her make-up and big dangling earrings and necklace. Poor Cathie got the shock of her life and began to cry. The children ran out into the lobby to see why their Mammy was crying, and Cathie told the boys that their Granda had died. Then Ellen left saying that she had to go up the road and inform Margaret of Granda's death. Before she left, Ellen asked Cathie if it would be alright for her to go to the dancing the next night, as it was Doctor Crock and his Crackpots, who were on. Cathie was angry, and said, "You cannot go to the dancing when your father had just died". Ellen replied, "What harm will it do him", but she did not go, because her old Aunties were down at the house to pay their respects.

The next, day after finding it hard to sleep the night before, and still feeling very tired, Cathie got up early and got the children ready and gave them breakfast before taking them down to Granda's house. Granda's corpse was laying in the coffin in his bedroom. Cathie and Margaret would not let the younger children go in. Jim took Jackie in and told him that they would have to kneel down and say a wee prayer for Granda. Jackie was frightened and was about to run out, when Jim shouted at him, "Don't be scared, are you a big wain ? A big feerty ? Look at me, I can go up and touch his face". But Jackie took fright and ran out of the room, and then Jim got a funny feeling, and ran out shortly after him. Big John and Margaret said that they were going home, and they asked Cathie if she would like to go up the road with them. As Granda's wee house was full of friends and relatives, Cathie thought that it would be a good idea to take the children home.

Cathie, Margaret and Big John returned early on the morning of the funeral with their children. Cathie and Margaret prepared the sanswiches and laid on a nice spread for the mourners as they returned from the cemetery.

The children got fed-up, so Jim and Jackie took them along to the park to let them play on the swings Cathie and Margaret told the two older boys to keep watch on the younger children. "Keep your eyes on them all the time, and don't let them wander off." Jim and Jackie turned their backs for a minute to give Thomas and Frankie a push on the swings, and when they turned round there was no sign of wee Patricia.

Jim asked Kathleen, as he panicked, "Where is wee Patricia ? Where has she gone ? She was standing beside you".

"Wee Patricia has gone missing, she has wondered off. What are we going to do ?" Jim asked Jackie in a state of near panic. "My Mammy will kill me. I only let her out of my sight for a minute. She was there one minute and gone the next". Jim said all twitching and shakey, the way he got when anything like that happened. We will have to start looking. Jim and Jackie took the younger children by the hand and went on a search, looking in all the backcourts, and up and down all the closes as they went along the street. Jim and a search party of children on one side of the street and Jackie and another group of children on the other. As time went by Jim began to feel physically ill. Wee Patricia was nowhere to be seen. Jim said to Jackie, "There is only one thing for us to do now, we will have to go back to Granda's house and tell my Mammy, and I'm dreading that, God knows what she will do when she hears what has happened."

The children arrived back at Granda's house and chapped the door, and as there was so many people in the house the children had to chap the door many times before someone heard them knocking and opened it. Jim shouted out as soon as he entered the living room, "Wee Patricia is missing, she has gone off. It was not my fault. I just turned my back for a minute, and she was gone". Poor Cathie was "up to high doe" with worry. The adults got up a search party and went out to look for Wee Patricia. They looked in all the backcourts up and down the closes in gardens and railway sidings and round behind old air-raid shelters. After some considerable time Cathie and the rest of the searchers became increasingly concerned and were about to inform the police. As Cathie walked along the street with tears in her eyes, her tears of sorrow turned to tears of joy as she looked up, and in the distance she could see a woman walking along the street, coming towards her, and she had wee Patricia by the hand. As they met, Cathie bend down and kissed and hugged wee Patricia, who was dirty and crying. Cathie asked her what had happened to her and where she had been. Patricia said that she was fed-up in the swing park and wanted home, but all the closes looked the same, and she didn't know Granda's close, and walked on and on. Cathie said to the woman, "I can't thank you enough, it was so good of you to bring my wee daughter back", and repeated, "Thank you, thank you", over and over again. The woman said that she recognized wee Patricia, as she had seen her with her family going down to visit her Granda many times.

After they had sat with May and Ellen mourning the death of their Da, Cathie and Margaret decided that it was time to take the children home.

Chapter Fourteen
To Kiss A Tear

About six months later Cathie's wages from Jimmy's merchant navy pay did not arrive, and she though that the post was at fault. She had something put by for a rainy day that she could use until the money arrived. The post may be late, she thought. Next week came, and there were no wages in the post, and into the third week there was no more money left. There was nothing, she told her sister, "I will have to go to the Social Security again and go through that humiliating experience again, I hate going to that place, but what else can I do?"

It was getting near Christmas 1957 and there was still no news of Jimmy. Cathie was worried about not having enough money to buy her kids Christmas presents. To make matters worse, Jim went into the living room one morning and took the cover off the budgie's cage and the poor wee bird was laying dead at the bottom of the cage, on its back with its legs sticking up in the air. The children were very sad. It was a problem for Cathie and Jim. "Take the bird out of the cage", Cathie said to Jim. "I don't like touching birds when they are alive, and I'm not going to touch it when it's bead." "Can you not get it Mammy" asked Jim. "I don't like touching it either" said Cathie, adding "Get a cloth and lift it out". "I can't". I can't and you can't, or wont lift the bird out of the cage, so you will have to go up the hill and ask Big John if he will come down and take Joey out and bury him in the garden". So Jim went up and got Uncle John to lift the budgie out of the cage and put him in a box, and then Jim took him out and dug a wee hole and buried him in the front garden.

"Let's cheer ourselves up, its getting near Christmas," Jim said as he came in from the garden after burying poor wee Joey. "That's a good idea Jim" said Thomas. Jim went into the cupboard in the lobby and at the back of the bottom shelf he found the box of decorations and the fairylights. He took the box of decorations into the living-room and his two wee sisters faces lit-up with jay as they saw the brightly coloured decorations for the tree and around the living-room. "We haven't any drawing pins to put up the decorations, I will have to go up to the shop and buy some, and what about a tree? We have got fairy lights, and there is a plug on them" said Jim. Jim took the lights out of their box and laid them on the floor, and put the plug into the socket in the wall. "They are not working!" The little sisters looked on excitement on their faces, a joy for Cathie to see. Then Kathleen and Patricia's faces got sad when the lights did not work. "There is a spare light bulb in the box" said Cathie. She took the spare light bulb and tried it round the set of twelve lights, and by stroke of luck, she got them to work. The two wee sisters and Thomas cheered and clapped their hands as they sat on the floor watching. "Thank God, they are still working", Cathie shouted, forgetting for a second about her financial situation: "Go up to the shop, Jim and get a Christmas Tree". "Can we afford it, Mammy ?" Jim asked as he was putting his hand out for the money. Jim went up to the shop and returned with a medium sized tree and took a bucket out into the backcourt to put earth in it to hold the tree upright. He put the tree on the table at the living-room window and with the assistance of his Mammy and the younger children, who handed the decorations up from the floor, he decorated it. Last, they put on the fairy-lights on and them switched on. It looked lovely. Then, Cathie got the ladders out and she put up the decorations across the ceiling and around the walls. "I will have to try and get something nice for the Christmas dinner, and we will have our Christmas dinner after Santa comes, and we have been to Mass to see the Baby Jesus in the crib," she told the children. Cathie was still worried about having enough money left to buy the children a good Christmas present. Each night as she went to bed Cathie knelt down by the side of her bed and prayed that something would come up, and that she would get some help.

Some days later the naval chaplain arrived at the house, and he has news of Jimmy. He told her that Jimmy had been at the atom bomb tests on Christmas Island, and he was now in hospital in Singapore, waiting to be sent home, and he gave Cathie some of the wages that Jimmy had due to him. When he heard what Cathie had gone through, he brought some presents for the children. Cathie thanked the chaplain as he handed her her share of Jimmy's wages from the merchant navy, and she was nearly in tears as she knew that her prayers had been answered, and her children would have a good Christmas after all. He told her that Jimmy would be sent home at the earliest convenience. Cathie and her children had a lovely happy, holy and contented Christmas. Thomas and the two wee sisters woke very early on Christmas morning. Kathleen and wee Patricia were really too young to realize what was happening. But, they were ecstatic with happiness as they walked hand and hand into the living room and saw the presents under the tree. They did not know what to do. "They are presents for you. Santa Thomas helped them to open up the parcels, as they thought that the girls were taking too long. Kathleen and Patricia were delighted with their identical dolls and the other wee gifts that Santa had left. Then Jim and Thomas opened their presents. Thomas got a garage and cars, and some other small presents, and Jim received books and writing equipment. However, Jim felt sadness as there was no present for his Mammy. "I feel terrible, there is no present for you", adding, "I would have bought you something if I had the money". Cathie replied, "Don't worry about that, Jim, Christmas is a time for children."

They got ready for breakfast, before going up the road to the chapel for Christmas Day morning Mass, and to see the baby Jesus in the crib. As they came out of the chapel they met Margaret and her boys, who had also been to Mass. The chapel was packed with the congregation attending Christmas Day Mass, and they also met some of their neighbours and their children. All the children were so excited as they told each other what Santa had brought them, and Cathie was so glad that her children had not been left out of the celebrations. Margaret and her boys came down to Cathie's house and Ellen brought some small gifts from each of the children from May and herself. May and Big John had to go to work, as they did not get a holiday on Christmas Day. The children played with there presents, and the younger children played more with the packaging. It had been a very long day for them and after the Christmas dinner, the younger children Kathleen, Patricia and Brian began to get very tired and fell asleep playing with their toys. Their Mammies put them all to bed, and Margaret took her two eldest boys home with Big John, who had come in from his work to see how they had all enjoyed their Christmas, and to see what Santa had brought the children.

After Christmas was over, Cathie looked forward to a nice quiet Hogmanay, and a happy and peaceful Ne'erday. As the time was approaching midnight Cathie said to Jim, as they sat watching the television in the livingroom, the younger children were in their beds (fast a sleep), "Jim, let's go to our beds". Jim asked if he could stay up to hear the bells and the ships on the River Clyde blowing their funnels, and Cathie agreed. After the clock struck midnight and the new year had began, Cathie said a quiet prayer that God would be good to them this year and bless them with good health and happiness. A short time later the door bell rang, and Cathie went to answer the door. It was Cissy and Peter from next door to wish them a Happy New Year. Cathie invited them in, and after a short time they asked her if she would like to go into a party in their house, but Cathie told them that she could not go and leave her children, but thanked them for their invitation.

One month into the new year, Jimmy arrived home unannounced. A taxi drew up at the close and he got out and walked up the path and into the close and rang the door bell. Cathie, who was in the children's bedroom changing the beds, shouted to Jim, "See who's at the door". Jim, who was in a happy frame of mind at the time went down the lobby, singing, or trying to, at the pitch of his voice, opened the door, and was struck speechless, when he saw his Daddy standing there. Jimmy came in, he walked straight passed Jim without saying a word, and Jim thought that he seemed like a stranger with his strange quiet manner. Jimmy walked straight passed him and up the lobby and into the livingroom, and sat down in his favourite armchair by the fire and put his large suitcase that he had bought down by the side of the chair. Cathie came into the livingroom and asked Jimmy what had happened to him. He could not give her an answer. Jim said to Jimmy, "Did you get your library book changed ?" adding that it was a long way to go to change a library book. Jimmy did not answer him, which Jim thought unusual. Jimmy opened his suitcase and brought out gifts for Cathie and the children.

A musical jewel box for Cathie, with a ballet dancer. The two daughters got silk kimonos, a toy car for Thomas and painting by numbers for Jim, which was really for himself. However, he did not bring any money. Cathie asked him again, but Jimmy could not, or would not say. The younger children, Thomas especially, were glad to see their Daddy home, Cathie had mixed feelings, but was glad he was safe, and asked him again what had happened to him, but Jimmy could not, or would not say.

After being home for sometime, Jimmy was still behaving very strangely. This worried Cathie, as it was having an adverse effect on the children. Cathie asked him if he was going to register for work and try to find a job, but he showed no interest in going out to find employment. Cathie tried to talk him out of it, to talk him round to going out with her and the children, and to take a pride in his appearance, but he was just not interested. Cathie went down to the doctor to discuss Jimmy's illness, and the doctor decided to give him medication and keep him "on the sick", as Jimmy had lost interest in everything, except his painting by numbers, that he had brought back for Jim.

As Jimmy's behaviour became stranger, members of Cathie's family and Jimmy's family came up to visit to try and talk him out of his depression. It was no use, he would not let the children turn up the volume on the wireless or the television. It caused a lot of animosity between father and son, Jimmy and Jim never did get on, and this situation got worse by the day. Jim turned the volume up, Jimmy turned it down, Jim turned it up again, and Jimmy turned it down so low that they could not hear a thing. This led to big fights and a lot of arguing, and it was beginning to tell on the health of the rest of the family. Cathie was beginning to lose a lot of weight with worrying about the effect that all this was having on the younger children. Jimmy would get up during the night and wander about the house wakening Cathie and the children up from their sleep. Poor Cathie was a "bag of nerves", as she said to Jimmy, "What is wrong with you ? Why are you behaving like this ?" but, she could not get a reasonable answer. Cathie went up to see the parish priest, and asked him to pray for her and the family. She told him that she was at her wits end, and that she did not know which way to turn.

One night Jim wakened up to find Jimmy wandering about the house semi-nude. He had no underpants on, pulling his vest down to cover his private parts. He was only going into the kitchenette for a drink of water, but Jimmy's manner was very strange, and he frightened Jim. Jim could not get back to sleep and when he went to school the following day he could not concentrate on his work in the various classes during the day. It was while in the history class that with the heat and with Jim being so over-tired he fell fast asleep. At the end of the lesson they tried to waken him up, and the other boys on finding that he was still asleep, decided to carry him up the stairs to another class for the next lesson. The teacher was most annoyed. He decided to take Jim to the headmasters office. The headmaster questioned Jim at great length about what time he went to bed, what television programmes he views, and his home life. He noted that Jim was shakier than usual, but he did not give him the strap on this occasion.

Mr. Richie, the headmaster could sense that there was something wrong, and he gave Jim a letter to take home to his parents. This really worried Jim, and he told his pals, Pat and the other Pat, "I'm in real trouble now, serious trouble, especially with my old man". As he got off the school bus and walked up the road, he thought about throwing the letter away and saying that he had lost it. Having maintained his common sense, he decided to keep the letter and give it to his Mammy. As he got to the door and rang the bell, he could feel his stomach begin to turn, and a dryness in his throat, and his hands began to shake more than usual. He handed the letter to Cathie, who read it at once. To Jim's relief Cathie was not angry, and she did not show the letter to Jimmy, as she knew that Jim was having a really hard time of it, with the way things were at home, with lack of sleep, and having to cope with Jimmy's illness, and also with the trouble with the boys at school. She told Jim, "Don't worry about it, I will go down and see the headmaster and explain the situation at home to him."

One evening, Jimmy stood up and announced that he was putting on his coat and going out for a breath of fresh air. "It's an awful night, it's cold and it's getting dark and beginning to rain". Cathie could not persuade him to stay in. Jim said, "Are you going to the library to change your book again ?" and he continued, "It was Hong Kong the last time you went to the library, where are you off to this time Cape Town ?" "You be quiet", Cathie shouted at Jim as Jimmy put his coat on and went out, saying, "I won't be long".

"Great", Jim said to Thomas, "We can turn up the sound on the telly, and open the curtains wide." Cathie was worried, but she did not want to show her concern to the children. It was back to the old anxiety for her of sitting and watching the clock and wondering if Jimmy would arrive home sober or drunk, or even arrive home at all. The hours passed by and she had to go to her bed. It was another night of tossing and turning as she could not sleep. After a long night came daylight, and Cathie was so very tired, but she had to get up to attend to the needs of her children. Wee Patricia had been sick again, and Cathie had to ask a neighbor if she could go and telephone the doctor and ask him if he could make a home visit.

Dr. Smith arrived at the house a few hours later. After he had gone into see wee Patricia, who was laying in her cot, very lifeless. Cathie told Dr. Smith that wee Patricia had been vomiting. He gave her a prescription for someone to take to the chemist. Dr. Smith then asked Cathie how she was keeping herself, as he noticed that she was looking very tired, and was losing a lot of weight. He also gave her a prescription for a tonic, and pills for Jim's nerves. Cathie told Dr. Smith that her two other children were fine, and did not seem to be affected by the disruption at home. She then said to Dr. Smith "I'm very worried about Jimmy, and I'm increasingly worried about his safety.

After a few days, wee Patricia began to "pick-up a little", she had become more active and was playing with the other children. She was beginning to eat some of her meals. Margaret came down to visit every day with her younger boys. May and Ellen also made visits to see how Cathie was coping, and see if they could offer any help. There was still no news of Jimmy, members of his family also visited to see if there was any news. Jim said to them, "He will probably be sailing the ocean waves".

Some days later there was a knock at the door. Cathie said to Jim, "I've got an awful feeling that that is the police at the door", and Jim replied, "I will come to the door with you Mammy, in case there is any bad news, I mean any news". They both hurried down the lobby, and Cathie opened the door. It was the police, and they asked if they could come in. Cathie showed them into the livingroom, and she was fearing the worst, that something had happened to Jimmy this time, although the police had been to her door a few times before. "He is alive", they told her, and he is in a mental hospital, and they continued to tell Cathie and

Jim that he had been living rough, and was found wandering. "You will have to go down and collect him", they told Cathie. "I can not go now, as I will have to make arrangements for someone to look after and feed my children. That will take sometime, as I am not on the telephone", Cathie replied.

After the police left Cathie and Jim were very worried about the state of mind that they might find Jimmy in. "I will go with you", Jim told his Mammy. Jim went up the road to ask Margaret if she would look after the younger children. It was a cold, very foggy day, as Cathie got the children ready and put the two young sisters in the go-chair, and with the boys by her side, they made their way up the hill to Margaret's house. Cathie told Margaret about the police coming and what had happened. Margaret felt very sorry for her sister, as she heard the story, and said to Cathie, "You are having an awful time of it. When will it ever end, its just one thing after another. Surely your luck will change." "Oh, I do hope so, Margaret, I can't take much more of this, I'm at my wits end, I could run away if it wasn't for my wains. I could never leave my wains, I love them so much", Cathie said. Cathie and Jim then left for a journey into the unknown.

As they left Margaret's house and made their way down to the bus stop, the weather was turning for the worst. It was getting colder and foggier, it was beginning to turn into a freezing fog as they waited and waited for the bus, which they thought would never come. After nearly one hour the bus arrived and they got on, and made the first leg of their journey as they sat shivering.

After the first bus ride into the city centre, they had to go and change onto another bus to continue their journey, out to the hospital in the countryside. After a second long bus journey, it was foggy and daylight was fading. As they walked through the main gates of the hospital, Cathie and Jim had to walk up a long eerie country lane, which had thick bushes and tall trees on either side. There was the occasional odd looking person walking up and down the lane. Jim said to his "I don't like the look of these people. I feel frightened". Cathie replied, "They are just poor sick people, and they won't do you any harm". Cathie did not want to admit that she was frightened too.

They were glad when they reached the main entrance to the hospital, where the lights were on. There were also some other visitors standing around. They made their way in and enquired directions to Jimmy's ward. Cathie asked to see him, and the staff nurse told her that he was not there and directed them to the psychiatrist's office.

Cathie knocked the door, and a quite spoken voice called "come in". They entered the dimly lit room. There was an old man sitting at his desk, with only a desk lamp on, and another small light. He did not ask them to sit down. Cathie and Jim stood in front of his big desk during their interview. The psychiatrist looked at them over his half-rimmed spectacals, and informed them that Jimmy was not there at the moment., Cathie was in despair. Had they gone all that way for nothing ? He went on to explain that Jimmy had been at the hospital but had walked out. On hearing this Cathie was most up-set. He then asked Jim how old he was. Jim informed him that he was fourteen, and the psychiatrist said that he was old enough to understand what he was about to tell them. He then proceeded to tell them that Jimmy had schizophrenia, and then he went on to explain, who gets schizophrenia, what causes it, what the symptoms are, and the treatment. Cathie and Jim were speechless when they were told this at first. Then Cathie asked him how they could help Jimmy, what could they do ?

Cathie and Jim returned to Margaret's house to collect the children. As soon as they went in the door Margaret said to Cathie and Jim, "come into the kitchenette, and I'll make you something to eat and a nice hot cup of tea, you must be freezing". Cathie and Jim ate the hot meal, which Margaret had prepared for them, and they enjoyed every bite, as they were feeling so hungry. Cathie told Margaret about the visit to the hospital, and what they had been told, and that she was frightened for the future. "That's terrible, I only wish that we could do more to help you." Margaret told Cathie as Cathie and Jim left and took the younger children home to their own house.

Some days passed, and there was no news of Jimmy. "He'll have gone to Hong Kong again, maybe to look for his library book" Jim said with a laugh. "It's no laughing matter, I'll have to go and see about getting money again, and I'm not looking forward to that." Cathie told Jim.

Quite late one Friday night the door bell rang. Cathie had just got Kathleen and Patricia bathed and into their cot and bed for the night, and was just finishing drying Thomas in the bathroom. The door bell rang, "I don't like answering the door at this time of night." Everytime the door-bell rung for the last two weeks Cathie's heart missed a beat. During that time Cathie had visits from her own family and Jimmy's.

This time Cathie had a feeling that it was Jimmy at the door. She and Jim went down the lobby. "I'll come with you Mammy, just in case it's him". Jim was genuinely frightened. The door bell rang again, and again. "Who is there, who is there" shouted Cathie. "It's me, Jimmy, open up, open up, open up" he shouted through the letter box. Still frightened Cathie and Jim opened the door. Standing there in front of them was Jimmy, who looked like an old tramp. He looked as if he had been sleeping rough, his clothes were dirty and smelly. He told them that he had been sleeping rough, and that God had looked after him. When Cathie heard this she knew that he was not his normal self. She told him to come in and go straight into the bathroom and strip off his dirty smelly clothes, and Jim took them out in the midden in the backcourt. Jimmy them got into the bath and gave himself a right good scrub, and washed his hair. Cathie went and got him fresh clothes. He got out of the bath and dried himself and put on the nice clean clothes.

"Go into the livingroom and sit by the fire to heat yourself up, and I will bring you a hot meal to heat you up" Cathie told him. They did not ask him any questions until after he had eaten, and he had a big warm mug of tea. "A mug for a mug" Jim thought, "Oh this will be good, I can't wait until he tries to explain this latest little episode", said Jim. "The man is ill, he needs our help", Cathie shouted at Him. Who replied, "You would think it was my fault, the way you are carrying on." After he had finished his meal, Cathie tried to get Jimmy to tell her what had happened to him. He could not, or would not tell her.

The next morning Cathie arranged for the doctor to make a house-call. "Oh Dr. Smith, you never seen to be away from this house, it's just one thing after another", Cathie told the doctor. But at least, she got a sick line from the doctor, and she would be sure of getting her sick-pay.

As the weeks went by, Jimmy's behavior became intolerable. "He won't let me open the curtains someday's" Cathie told Margaret and Big John when she went up to see them. "I would leave, but with four children, I have nowhere to go, and who would take me in with four children ?" said Cathie. "You will have to look after your own health for the sake of your children, your weight is down to just six stones" Margaret told her, and went on, "Go and ask if you can get a house of your own. See the doctor or the priest". Cathie said, "If I go and get a house of my own, he will just come and annoy me, and there are a lot of women in the same situation with their husbands through drink or gambling etc. Cathie, however did agree to go and seek help.

Cathie went home and thought about her chat with Margaret. She was worried about her own health and what would happen to her children if she took ill and taken into hospital. Her mind was in a turmoil she did not no what to do for the best. One night she went up to see the parish priest, and talk over her problems with him. Life was becoming unbearable. Jimmy would not let the children turn up the volume on the television, or open the curtains.

It was getting late, and the children and Cathie had all gone to sleep in the front bedroom, as Jimmy was acting strange, saying he could hear voices. Cathie and the children felt very frightened as they could hear Jimmy going up and down the lobby shouting to himself. Jim pushed a chest of drawers against the bedroom door. Then Cathie said to Jim, "Well, that's it, I've had enough, I can't take anymore". Jim and Cathie got the children up and dressed. Jim opened the front bedroom window and managed to squeeze the small go-chair through and held it until it slid down the wall on to the ground in the garden. They then got a chair by the window, and Jim climbed out, Cathie handed the children out, one by one to Jim, who was shaking like a leaf, but knew that he had a job to do. He put his two young sisters into the go-chair and told Thomas to hold on to the side. Then Cathie climbed out of the window, and closed it behind her. It was a cold, wet and dark windy night, and the children were scared as the wind blew through the trees. "That's it", Cathie told Jim "We are away now and we are definitely not going back." Jim replied, "I hope you mean it this time." To which she replied "I really do. No way am I going back to that house."

They arrived at Margaret's house soaking wet, with only the clothes they stood in. Margaret got them dried off and they squeezed into beds with Margaret's boys.

The following day wee Patricia became ill, and they sent for the doctor in the morning. The following day her condition was slightly worse. Cathie said to Margaret, "Please go and telephone the doctor again. I'm becoming very concerned about her". The doctor arrived an examined her, and gave her another prescription for her to try. The next evening Cathie and Margaret become more anxious about wee Patricia's health, and asked Big John to go out and telephone for an ambulance to take wee Patricia to the hospital. Jim sat in the big fireside chair, by the side of the big coal fire in Margaret's livingroom with wee Patricia on his knee. The heat and light from the flames in the fire shone onto wee Patricia's face. The only other light in the room was the light coming from the small lamp on top of the television. She did not cry, she just lay in Jim's arms looking up and occasionally going into a wee sleep. Jim knew that she was very ill, and there was hardly any weight in her small body. As he cradled her in his arms he thought he could hear the "death rattle", that he had heard the adults talk about years ago. Tears filled his eyes, as he had a thought, a feeling that if wee Patricia goes away she might die and he may not see her again. A tear from his eye dropped down onto wee Patricia's cheek, and Jim bent down to kiss a tear, and his wee sister that he might never see again.

The ambulance arrived. It was very cold, as there was no heating on. Cathie got into the ambulance with wee Patricia cradled in her arms accompanied by Margaret. Jim watched from the window as the ambulance pulled away and vanished down the road until it was out of sight. All the other children were in their beds sleeping, and Big Uncle John told Jim to go to his bed too. Jim replied that he could not go to his bed and sleep until he knew how wee Patricia was, but to satisfy Uncle John he went into the room and lay down, but he could not sleep.

Some hours later Cathie and Margaret arrived back from the hospital. By this time it was near the middle of the night. As they came in the door they were crying. Jim heard them and jumped up and as he was about to go out of the room, Cathie came in and told him that wee Patricia was dead. She had died in the ambulance just as they had reached the hospital. The doctor on duty told them, "If this child had arrived at the hospital one hour earlier, we could have saved her life."

The following day Big John had to go down and tell Jimmy, and they were worried about how he would take the news of wee Patricia's death. He came up and he cried too. He asked Cathie to go back. Cathie told him no, as it would be no life for her remaining children. Auntie May agreed, and some days later Cathie hired a removal van and took some of the furniture and the children's toys and clothes, and her washing machine, after all, "it was a present", she said. They left more than half the furniture and the television. Cathie locked the door for the last time, and went to join Jim in the removal van. As the van drove off and out of the avenue they were off to another new beginning.

About the Author

I was employed in mechanical engineering, and I am on the management committee of the housing association and served on sub-committees including finance, staffing and appeals. Also Chairman of WestWorks Ltd. And Scotinch Services Ltd which I do voluntary to assist my community and create local employment.

I attended a special school for handicapped children, and clinics for physiotherapy. I worked at a publishers , then an engineering course at The National Spastics Society training centre, then worked in commercial vehicle manufacturing.

My interest are varied: local, national and international politics. Computing and video production, theatre, cinema , reading and writing.

I have cerebral palsy and have been married for thirty years with one daughter. I participated in a television programme produced in my home about tenement refurbishment . And also featured an interview with me about my writing. I also appear on a DVD production for Community Scotland - Wider Action.

My manuscripts are: the trilogy SHAKING / HEAD-BOY / STILL SHAKING my series of children's books: THE ENCHANTED NURSERY featuring: NESSIE'S FRIENDS / HEATHER AND HAMISH / PERCY PENGUIN / REGGIE RABBIT / FUN IN FLORIDA. Other writing pursuits are: JIMMY full-length comedy-drama screenplay A GOOD MOVE thirty minute comedy, HEATHER AND HAMISH short screenplay of children's story - all are adaptations from my manuscripts, and "SHOULD WE STILL GO?" short play/screenplay toi illustrate the diversity of my writing.

My registered copyright and trademark at Companies House are: Jim Higgins all rights reserved Higgiland Enterprises I have suggestions/recommendations for commercial and enterprise in relation to my books and screenplays, and MY SHAKING HANDS productions.

Jim Higgins, Higgiland Enterprises

OTHER BOOKS BY
JIM HIGGINS:

Head Boy
Still Shaking

THE ENCHANTED NURSERY SERIES:

Nessie's Friends
Percy Penguin's Friends
Reggie Rabbit at the Seaside
Fun in Florida
Heather and Hamish
The Tartan Dolls' Edinburgh Castle Adventure

www.ingramcontent.com/pod-product-compliance
Lightning Source LLC
Chambersburg PA
CBHW031320290526
45784CB00014B/298